Latino Folk Medicine

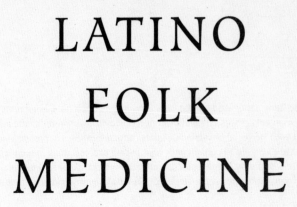

LATINO
FOLK
MEDICINE

**Healing Herbal Remedies
from Ancient Traditions**

ANTHONY M. DeSTEFANO

Ballantine Books • New York

A Ballantine Book
Published by The Ballantine Publishing Group
Copyright © 2001 by Anthony M. DeStefano

All rights reserved under International and Pan-American Copyright Conventions. Published in the United States by The Ballantine Publishing Group, a division of Random House, Inc., New York, and simultaneously in Canada by Random House of Canada Limited, Toronto.

www.randomhouse.com/BB/

Library of Congress Catalog Card Number: 00-110327

ISBN 0-345-43836-1

Manufactured in the United States of America

Designed by Ann Gold

First Edition: February 2001

10 9 8 7 6 5 4 3 2 1

Latino Folk Medicine

Introduction

In an apartment in the East Harlem section of Manhattan, a diminutive, stout woman with closely cropped hair looked with concern at the small boy in the brass bed. The child was covered with a thick layer of blankets and was trying to rest as best he could despite the fact that breathing was made difficult by an infection in his lungs.

The time was around 1927—an era when doctors still made house calls—and the visiting physician seated at the bedside turned to the woman and told her that it would be best if the boy got plenty of rest. He also told her to get some mustard seeds and do what she knew from the old country: work the plant material with water into a paste and place the entire plasterlike concoction onto a thick towel. The wet cloth was to be placed on the little boy's chest for a few minutes. If all went well, the mustard plaster would dilate the blood vessels in his chest and bring in more blood circulation, breaking up the congestion and clearing the child's bronchial tubes and lungs.

The woman standing by the bed was my Italian immigrant grandmother. The little boy laid low with bronchitis was my father.

Of course, my father made a full recovery and went on to

grow up in a part of New York City that was then a center of Italian and Jewish immigrants. Today, the area where my family established its roots in the United States is still a center of immigration and still a place where folk medicine is practiced. But the old European community has moved on and been replaced by a migration from Latin America, a massive flow of Spanish-speaking peoples that has reshaped the political and social landscape of the city.

The old tenement where my family lived is now a vacant shell of a building. But much of the neighborhood, still with its share of old housing stock, is alive and vibrant, resonating with the sounds, sights, and smells of Hispanic culture. In the years after World War II, Puerto Ricans arrived in large numbers. Though not technically immigrants—their homeland is a commonwealth of the United States—Puerto Ricans gave East Harlem a distinctive barrio flavor. With an infrastructure of Latino bodegas, churches, and stores, the area became a magnet for other Spanish-speaking immigrants, so much so that by the 1990s large sections of the neighborhood were home to Dominicans, Ecuadorians, Mexicans, and others of Latin heritage.

By the year 2001, the Hispanic immigrant population is projected to be the largest minority group in New York City. Looking to the rest of the country, Hispanics are expected to grow by the year 2025 to forty million.

Hispanics arriving in New York, Los Angeles, Houston, or any other major center of immigration bring with them many aspects of their traditional cultures. Among these are the traditional medicinal practices, known to Anglos by the more contemporary terms *complementary medicine* and *alternative medicine*. Based largely on the use of a wide variety of medicinal plants but tied to a number of other, more spiritual practices, Hispanic traditional medicine has been firmly transplanted along with the immigrant cultures. This is clearly evident in a walk through East Harlem today. Within a few blocks of my family's old tenement apartment on East 112th Street, where my grandmother practiced her Mediterranean folk cures, are a number of *botánicas*, shops that sell medicinal plants, perfumes, fragrant water, and other items used by Hispanics for health care and a variety of religious and spiritual purposes. The same types of stores are also found sprinkled throughout other city neighborhoods around the country where Hispanics live in large numbers.

Based on traditions that have been passed down through centuries from ancient Mayan, Aztec, and Inca cultures, as well as from the indigenous peoples of the Amazon and elsewhere in Latin America, Hispanic folk medicine is one of several cultural traditions relying on plants. No one knows for certain when humans began using plants to deal with illness, but it is a safe bet that it was sometime in the last ten thousand years, the period of time within which, botanists believe, plants began to be cultivated. The Chinese have a written medical text that talks of herbal remedies dating to 2000 B.C., while the ancient Ayurvedic practices of India are at least as old. The ancient Greek physician Hippocrates wrote of useful medicinal plants, as did the Roman physician Galen. In the first century A.D., Dioscorides, a doctor who traveled with the Roman army, wrote *De materia medica*, which describes nearly six hundred plants said to have healing powers, a work that is referred to even today as a classic in botanical and pharmacological history.

There are no extensive surviving written works encapsulating the medicinal knowledge of Hispanic cultures from

ancient times, however. There are some fragments of documents, but nothing that the cultures of Latin America could
rely on as an available written repository of the knowledge
of their traditional medical systems. Instead, more informal
means are used to transmit the traditions of Latin American
folk medicine down through generations. *Curanderos,* lay
healers who work with the spiritual elements of a patient
as a way of treating an illness, are one way the old traditions have been kept alive, particularly in Mexican culture.
Their healing gift is one that comes with years of training
and hands-on experience at curing the body and the soul
together. Shamans and other healers have also been trans-
mitters of this specialized knowledge of health care, particularly in the tropical forest areas. But for the most part it
has been the informal and intimate oral connections—
mothers talking to daughters, fathers to sons—that explain
how Hispanic traditional medicine has made its way down
through the centuries.

Today many more Americans are turning to alternative
medical practices. A study published in 1998 in the *Journal
of the American Medical Association* estimated that 42.1 percent of Americans used at least one of sixteen alternative therapies in the previous year, up from 33.8 percent
in 1990. The therapies most often encountered include
herbal medicine, massage, folk remedies, energy healing,
and homeopathy. It is estimated that herbal remedies, already a staple of the health care of many Latinos, are now
used by over thirty million people in the United States. A
walk through any supermarket or health food store will
reveal rows of shelves stocked with herbal nutritional products. In 1997, according to *Consumer Reports,* it was estimated that Americans spent over $12 billion for vitamins,

herbal supplements, and other health products. World-wide, the usage of herbal and other folk remedies is practiced by 80 percent of the human race, according to an estimate by the World Health Organization.

For most Americans using herbal supplements, attention has been focused on key botanical products such as saw palmetto, St. John's wort, kava kava, and ginkgo biloba. The roster of products continues to grow, even though legally they can be marketed only as nutritional supplements and not cures or drugs. Regardless of the Food and Drug Administration's position on the legality of using botanical substances as medicine, many Hispanics in the United States resort to medicinal plants as a regular way of coping with illness and will continue to do so as their tradition and experience dictate. Their list of herbal remedies ranges from the well-known aloe vera to the more obscure cana agria, or sour cane. It is a pharmacopoeia with hundreds of listings.

A large part of the folk reliance on plant-based remedies among Hispanics comes from the fact that their various places of origin in Latin America—Mexico, Central and South America, the Caribbean—are tropical areas with abundant plant life. Temperate areas such as the United States and Europe have impressive flora as well, but when it comes to plants that are loaded with healing possibilities, the tropics are a special case. As any botanist will point out, the plants in tropical regions live in intensely competitive environments, where cold weather does not eliminate the threat of insects and herbivorous animals and where fungi and other organisms flourish all year round. As a result, tropical plants produce chemicals that help them to survive. It is these chemicals that make the plants useful as folk medicines. It comes as no surprise that, living intimately over the centuries with such an abundant source of medicinal plants, Hispanic cultures developed a reliance on a system of herbal medicine.

The aim of this book is to familiarize the reader—both layperson and medical professional—with some of the most popular Latino folk cures based on plants. With the Spanish-speaking population continuing to grow in the United States, reaching an estimated thirty-two million in 2000, it is fair to say that some traditional medicines from the Latin cultures will move outside of the immigrant communities and become acceptable and useful to mainstream American culture. Often, conventional health care practitioners, be they doctors, psychiatrists, or other specialists, are unfamiliar with and dismissive of the traditional remedies used by immigrant cultures. One of the reasons for that, according to Elena Avila, a trained psychologist who is a practicing *curandera*, is that many physicians will not use a course of treatment that cannot be defined in a "linear, scientific approach." Most medical doctors, she said in her book *Woman Who Glows in the Dark*, believe that diseases and illness have specific causes (bacteria or viruses, for instance) instead of nonspecific causes, such as emotion and soul. While it may certainly be difficult for a doctor steeped in Western science to embrace the spiritual elements of Hispanic medicine, knowledge of the health practices and beliefs valued by a culture can go a long way in helping a physician tend to an immigrant's needs by improving communication and even making conventional medicine a more available option when it is needed in the case of a serious illness.

There is another reason for exploring the traditional

medicines of the Hispanic cultures, and that has to do with preservation of a special knowledge that is at risk of being lost. Other writers have dealt with the point more extensively, particularly botanists and other scientists who fear that the earth's rain forests and the indigenous cultures they support are endangered. But, simply put, folk traditions are fragile, and with the passing of each generation we lose a little of the human store of knowledge. "The pharmaceutical use of many plant species—rosy periwinkle, aspirin, ipecac, curare and quinine among many others—have long histories of indigenous use," writes botanist Michael Balick of the New York Botanical Garden, "but more of this knowledge disappears with the passing of each generation of native healers." While studying medicinal plants in the Central American nation of Belize, Balick and his colleagues came across a number of cases where a grandchild of a healer lamented never having learned the ways of traditional Latino medicine when those who had that special knowledge were alive. This book strives to serve a purpose in the preservation of such knowledge.

While use of plants and plant substances in Latino health traditions is clearly an emphasis here, this book is not meant to be blind advocacy for or an uncritical look at some of the practices. Even a cursory look at some of the medical literature will show cases where use of some herbal products, as well as reliance on folk healers, is believed to have resulted in illness or death. So, where needed, there are cautions and warnings about some of the plants and folk practices described.

Widespread as the use of medicinal plants may be, there have not been many human clinical trials with the substances to test their effectiveness and safety. Simply put, clinical trials are an expensive proposition, running into the tens of millions of dollars, and are undertaken in this country by drug companies only when there is a strong likelihood that a product will pass governmental muster and find its way to the consumer market. However, there is a great deal of study into the medicinal uses of plants in laboratory settings, using either human cells in a test tube or petri dish (known as in vitro testing) or animals (in vivo), much of which will be explained in this book.

With advances in computer science and laboratory techniques, a number of pharmaceutical companies are conducting systematic searches in Latin America for plants that may provide new drugs. Some studies have confirmed that certain plant substances are not harmful and may in fact be capable of doing what practitioners of traditional medicine claim, laying the groundwork for more complex studies. Other results are more specifically promising, and have led to further studies, particularly in the areas of AIDS, diabetes, cancer, and Alzheimer's disease. Two medicinal plants highlighted in this book figure prominently in current medical research: cat's claw *(Uncaria tomentosa)* is being studied as the source of a possible drug to fight Alzheimer's disease, and dragon's blood *(Croton lechleri)* has proved useful in combating some of the problems associated with AIDS. But still other experiments have been unable to verify that the reputed properties of some medicinal plants used in Hispanic cultures exist. In fact, some of the plant products, as this book will show, may be dangerous for human consumption and should be avoided, despite the fact that they are still used.

Western medical tradition has taught us to rely on scientific methods to determine what medicines are useful to treat our ills. For the most part, that has served us well. But to examine the area of Hispanic traditional medicine requires a broader approach. Scientific testing, while an important part of medicine, has a tough time penetrating some aspects of medicinal treatments that are deeply embedded in the folk traditions. For instance, how can a scientist, so rooted in the empirical, grasp what Elena Avila means when she explains *curanderismo* as "medicine and spirituality practiced simultaneously"? It is this reliance on the spiritual that guides some of the health practices of Spanish-speaking immigrants.

A crucial spiritual element involved in Hispanic traditional medicine is that of *espiritismo*, an amalgam of beliefs prevalent in Puerto Rican communities. Known also as spiritism, the tradition is rooted in the belief that the spirit world and the material world coexist and interact. Readings of the spirit world are carried out by *mediunidades* (mediums) during individual *consultas* or in larger gatherings. At the gatherings or *consultas*, people are believed to gain insights into their psychological or physical maladies. The treatments in such cases may be herbal tonics or some spiritual act such as a blessing or anointment with a special oil.

Santería, widely reported on in the popular news media because of cultlike practices involving the ritual slaughter of animals, is also a religious element of some Hispanic cultures that has health care ramifications. Essentially a religion that blends the elements of Christianity with those of the African worship of several gods, Santería is a mixture of magic and religion. Its practices sometimes find their way into *espiritismo*, and in neighborhood *botánicas* the ritualistic elements of Santería—coconut shells, beaded necklaces, figurines of saints, and seashells—are found in abundance alongside the various herbal remedies.

So to understand the health traditions of the Hispanic immigrant communities in the United States requires more than a scientific look. It also requires an appreciation of the value those cultures place on the spiritual and the magical in the art of healing. While those elements have been closely intertwined with the practical in Latino cultures, they may not be something that the American mainstream culture can understand and accept as a viable health practice.

Healthwise, the Hispanic immigrant communities seem to follow the general trend for other newcomers. Studies show that upon arrival in the United States, immigrants generally tend to be young and healthy, although health professionals and government agencies also report that some who migrate do so to take advantage of Medicaid in order to have medical procedures that were just too risky, too expensive, or unavailable at home. Over time, studies show, the health of immigrants can deteriorate—a function, it seems, of increased fat intake and a general lack of access to quality health care. These trends have proven to be particularly punishing for Hispanics.

Studies done by the federal government as well as private researchers have found the Hispanic population in the United States historically to be suffering from poor access to health care. This in turn has affected the group's overall mortality and morbidity. In a study done by the *Journal of the American Medical Association*'s Council on Scientific Affairs in 1991, Hispanics were found to be spending more of their money on health care but were more likely to be unin-

sured than the rest of the country's population. Compared
with whites, twice as many Hispanics reported using hospital emergency departments as their source of primary care,
mainly because they were less likely to have private medical insurance. Public hospitals rarely provide continuity of
health care, according to the study. "Poverty and lack of
health insurance are the greatest impediments to health
care for Hispanics," the council's report concluded.

Poverty, coupled with cultural and language barriers, has
made reliance by Hispanics on traditional medicines more
essential for health care in the various Latino immigrant
communities. "The *botánicas* are the drugstores of the poor
people," says Jorge Vargas, proprietor of one such establishment in Manhattan. Similar remarks are also heard in
the marketplaces of Central America, where the high cost of
health care is a definite problem. But the people have their
yerba buena, the "good herb," and for many that makes a
big difference in their lives.

For years I viewed alternative medicine as something
practiced by people who wore tie-dyed clothing and san-
dals. However, the idea for this book came in one of those
strange yet wonderful moments when a door to one's imagi-
nation opens unexpectedly. I had worked on a *Newsday*
newspaper article that dealt, in summary fashion, with the
various folk medicinal practices such as acupuncture and
herbal medicines used by immigrants in New York City. I
did not expect to visit the subject again. But calls from
readers showed that there was a great deal of interest in the
alternatives we wrote about. Clearly the public is hungry for
news about medical practices that complement the existing
medical system. Looking around, I discovered that Hispanics use hundreds of herbs and plant materials for their

health care. In fact, the use ethnic communities make of plants, as either food or medicine, has spawned an entire scientific specialty known as ethnobotany, a term credited to the American botanist John W. Harsberger in the latter part of the nineteenth century. Clearly the subject is significant in the twenty-first century as well. Hence the idea for this book was born.

This work is meant to be an informative look at some of the medicinal plants used in the folk healing traditions of the various Hispanic cultures. There are literally thousands of such plants throughout Latin America—not an unreasonable amount considering that the overall number of plant species is estimated to be as high as eighty thousand in the Amazon region alone. Some are specific to certain locales. But others are used widely by Spanish-speaking peoples wherever they may be: from Tierra del Fuego, Argentina, to Pelham Bay, the Bronx. This book features sixty-three of the most widely known healing plants used by Hispanics, providing insight into their history and their traditional and modern uses, as well as medical evidence about their efficacy. Because all plants contain chemicals—known to scientists as phytochemicals—that can impact the human body and interact with other drugs, anyone contemplating using medicinal plants should consult a doctor first to avoid potential problems and adverse reactions. This caution will be repeated often in this book, and it is one always worth keeping in mind.

When Professor Daniel Moerman of the Department of Anthropology at the University of Michigan began work on his classic book about the herbal medicines used by the Indians of North America, he said, what he knew about plants was encompassed by the succinct phrase "green is up, brown is down." In the beginning of this book project my knowledge of plants was just as rudimentary. To gain insight into the wide variety of medicinal plants used by Hispanic immigrants required numerous visits to *botánicas* in New York City and to the New York Botanical Garden in the Bronx, as well as a visit to Costa Rica. Along the way, I talked with government officials, doctors, anthropologists, botanists, ethnobotanists, chemists, sociologists, and historians, including one specializing in Byzantine history. I spent hours with vendors of medicinal plants and the people who use them. It was a journey of discovery for me, always the best kind. It is a trip I am glad you also have decided to take.

Anthony M. DeStefano
New York, N.Y.
Fall 1999

CHAPTER ONE

The Spirit and the Medicine

Under the gaze of the ceramic saints on the shelves and the smiling Buddha by the door, a dark-haired, heavyset Dominican woman paced back and forth in the store. Looking out onto Broadway in upper Manhattan, she was clearly anxious; her animated eyes betrayed her inner turmoil.

The woman, named Lisa, spoke softly in Spanish to no one in particular as the store's proprietor, a quiet, bespectacled man named Antonio Mora, chatted with a visitor. Mora's establishment is known in Spanish as a *botánica*, a place where people can buy a variety of medicinal herbs, perfumed waters and oils, incense, and other items endowed with religious significance. Customers can also, for a small fee, talk with Lisa in a private *consulta*, a heart-to-heart talk that delves into the magical and the spiritual. An errant child, a marriage problem, depression, anxiety—Lisa is able to talk about all of it with visitors to the shop.

But on this particular day she was preoccupied with something more immediate. A man had appeared earlier outside the Botánica Santa Barbara and uttered some words to a large statue of Saint Barbara, the store's namesake, which was the centerpiece of the window display. No

one heard what the man said, but Lisa figured it had to be
nothing good. For he was reputed to be a *santero*, a practitioner of a Cuban-African religion that has many followers
in New York City's Hispanic community, and when he had
last been in the store he had not left on very good terms, at
least according to Mora.

"He stopped outside and talked to Santa Barbara," Mora
said, gesturing toward the large porcelain religious statue in
his store's window. "She saw him," Mora went on, referring
to Lisa. "The spirits told her something."

The spirits had apparently told Lisa something about the
negative forces the man had tried to use, and she knew she
had to act fast. She gathered up a glass bowl and some
items from behind the counter and disappeared into the
back room of the store, the place where she plies her own
trade. Mora, a soft-spoken man who had emigrated from
Cuba three decades earlier, seemed to have a slightly be-
mused smile as he watched Lisa go through her paces.
When she went to the back of the store, Mora turned to talk
with a visitor by a display counter stocked with piles of
herbs and plants.

Mora's *botánica* is well known in New York City. Located
near the George Washington Bridge, it is right in the heart
of New York's thriving Dominican community. Fed by a
steady stream of immigration, the area now has the largest
concentration of Dominicans outside their homeland. The
rush to open businesses catering to this immigrant culture
has been so steady that there is hardly a vacant storefront
along Broadway and the side streets. The neighborhood resembles other Latino ethnic enclaves in East Harlem, Los
Angeles, and Miami. Stores that once catered to an older

German community around World War II have been replaced by restaurants, boutiques, butcher shops, electronics stores, and Chinese restaurants, all sporting signs in Spanish. Remittance and telephone stores cater to a steady clientele who wire money back to the Dominican Republic, the economy of which is partly sustained by the flow of cash sent from immigrants living in New York.

Botánica Santa Barbara's niche is a special one for the city's Hispanic community and is symbolic of both the widespread use of medicinal plants and, as Lisa's presence reminds us, the reliance on spiritual elements and religion for health care among Latinos. No one knows for certain how many *botánicas* exist in New York, but where Hispanic populations settle, the *botánica* will soon follow. If none exists to serve the community, enterprising men and women will start selling medicinal plants and religious items from their apartments. If business improves, they may expand their operations to storefronts.

Each *botánica* is unique, but most stock the same things: magical perfumed air sprays, oils, votive candles, and religious figurines that relate to Roman Catholicism, Santería, and even Buddhism. There are commonplace medicines, such as Vicks, and more specialized ones known only to Hispanics, such as *siete jarabes*, or seven syrups, a blend of extracts from seven plants, including wild cherry and castor (used in Latin cultures as an expectorant for the treatment of asthma). Medicinal plants are also in abundance, perfuming the air with the smell of mint, chamomile, and many other types of vegetation.

Mora stores his medicinal herbs and plants in a refrigerated display case, which he believes keeps the products fresh. In other shops the herbs are kept out in the open, often in a helter-skelter array of boxes and crates. There is a steady turnover, said Mora. For no matter what other health care Hispanics may use, experts estimate that about half rely on folk medicines, a figure that remains constant even when education or employment status is taken into account.

It is not just Hispanics, Mora insisted, who come to the *botánica*. There is a substantial flow of traffic from other ethnic groups such as African-Americans and Asians.

"A lot of white people, a lot of people who spend money, come in here," he said, adding that he even attracts customers who work at the nearby Columbia-Presbyterian Medical Center, the largest hospital in the metropolitan area.

Having emigrated from Cuba shortly after Fidel Castro came to power, Mora landed in New York after a brief stay in Miami and began his career as a waiter, working in some of the big hotels. A couple of days a week Mora attends to the affairs of Botánica Santa Barbara, in which he took a part ownership after some friends approached him with the business proposition.

Mora does not pretend to know the science behind the medicinal plants. But he does know what sells and why people continue to buy. Waving his hand in front of the display case, Mora pointed out insulina, a plant that, as the name suggests, is used because it is believed to control diabetes, a disease that is particularly prevalent among Hispanics, according to federal government health studies. Ruda, known by the English name rue, is also a big seller and has been used in Latin America as everything from an abortifacient to a treatment for cancer and headaches, even though some experts say it can cause severe stomach pain, vomiting, and even death if taken internally. Also evident are herbs such as roma sarquey, used in Santería to clean up evil, Mora said.

As Mora was talking about the plants, Lisa emerged from the back room of the *botánica* holding a glass bowl of water colored blue with a dye that came in a small paper-wrapped cube. Floating in the liquid were clumps of camphor, a substance distilled from the wood of a tree and normally used as a liniment. But camphor is also known to be a disinfectant; combined with some ammonia Lisa had added, the water had an unusual potency against germs and, she hoped, against the evil that threatened the shop.

Walking to the front of the store, Lisa stopped by the door and with a paper cup began splashing the blue water onto the floor and throw rug that lay in front of the medicinal plants. Going behind the glass-topped counter, she splashed some more, making sure to cover the spots hidden near Mora's desk. When she was done, Lisa cleaned up the floor with a cloth mop, using long, languid strokes. She said nothing and returned to the rear of the *botánica*. Any prayers she may have spoken were internal ones, known only to her and the powers she addressed.

Lisa soon came back out again, carrying a coconut in a silver chalice. Asking Mora for a jar of palm oil, she then smeared some of the oil lengthwise along the coconut. Lighting a black candle and sticking it atop the oil-streaked coconut, Lisa walked the concoction over to the door and placed it on the floor next to a gilded porcelain statue of a smiling Buddha. She then went to the back of the shop again.

"It is to protect this place," Mora said about the ritual Lisa was performing.

Many *botánicas* have people like Lisa affiliated with

them, emblematic of the inseparable link that traditional medicine in the Hispanic community has with spiritual and religious components. Sickness is very often perceived to be not solely a question of microbes and biochemical causes but inextricably intertwined with the spiritual elements of a person's life and with those who take on the job of performing the healing. This is particularly true in the Puerto Rican community, which has deep historical ties to *espiritismo*. According to one survey of Puerto Rican households in New York, 53 percent of the families had at least one person who believed in *espiritismo*.

"Spiritism is the more traditional healing practice among Puerto Ricans," says Vivian Garrison, who did a medical anthropological study in the South Bronx in the late 1960s. "[But] in its present form and its literate tradition it dates back only to the last half of the nineteenth century and the writings of Alan Kardec."

An engineer and hypnotist, Kardec, known also by the pseudonym Hippolyte de Rivail, wrote about and gave form to the belief in spirits that was popular in Europe during the late nineteenth century. Some of the adherents to spiritism and Kardec's teachings were Victor Hugo, Mark Twain, and Napoleon III. In his *Book of the Spirits*, Kardec expounded upon a detailed system of relationships among spirits and the living beings, known as *seres*. It is a complex system of good, imperfect, and pure spirits, with various levels within levels. But the essential elements, according to Garrison, are *protecciones*, Catholic saints or Santería deities, and *mediunidades*, or mediums, who are able to communicate with helpful or good spirits. It is in the latter category that Lisa from the Botánica Santa Barbara seems to fit.

Spiritism seems more deeply entrenched in the Puerto Rican community than in any other Hispanic group. Beginning in the 1950s, Puerto Ricans set up a number of spiritual centers, known as *centros spirituales* or "white tables" because of a table covered by a white cloth at which twelve men known as "apostles" sat.

"Each apostle received a spirit for a case," remembers Jorge Vargas, a *botánica* owner in East Harlem, "and people came for healing. Each [apostle] would prescribe something, prayers, blessings, washing with herbs," as well as a decoction or bath with some kind of herbal remedy. The aim, according to Vargas, was to cure both psychological and physical ailments, which were often linked.

Vargas believes the spiritual centers helped a lot of Puerto Ricans in their time. Over the years they disappeared because they usually charged nothing for their services, he said. It remained then for individuals like Lisa, often working out of *botánicas*, to fill the need and work the spiritual cures that the community still pursues. While the ritual of the white table may be gone, the spiritual nature of many Hispanic healing practices remains evident.

There are two main ideas that need to be comprehended in order to understand the spiritual aspect of Hispanic folk medicine. According to a study of folk medicine in Puerto Rican communities done by Dr. Lee M. Pachter and others and published in the *Archives of Pediatric and Adolescent Medicine*, a traditional belief in Hispanic culture is that emotions can cause physical illness. For instance, it is thought that asthma, a common childhood malady, can be controlled by keeping the child calm, Pachter said. Maintaining balance, he stressed, is a key part of the Puerto Rican ethnomedical belief system. *Espiritismo* also holds that illness can be caused by disharmony or bad forces in a person's social relationships.

To treat illnesses, adherents of *espiritismo* not only will talk with mediums but will also bathe in water infused with medicinal plants, pray to various saints, or burn any one of a number of tall prayer candles that Mora and other *botánica* owners sell in great numbers. A number of illnesses, including some problems believed to be caused by spiritual or psychological disturbances, are tended to with herbal and plant remedies. A condition known as *susto*, or fright, which occurs following a frightening event, has as its symptoms anxiety and insomnia. It is often treated by Hispanic folk healers with the ritual passing of an egg over the patient, followed by the drinking of mint or herbal tea, which, particularly if chamomile is used, can have a calming and sedative effect. According to one study of Mexican folk remedies done at the Texas Tech University Health Sciences Center, colic, known as *cólico* among Hispanics, is also treated by mint and chamomile, as is *empacho*, the folk medicine term for a blocked intestine.

In his store, Mora sells plenty of chamomile and mint, both fresh and dried. But customers of Botánica Santa Barbara are also attracted to items that have no known biological effect on a person but are important elements of another part of the Hispanic ethnomedical system—Santería.

Santería (also known in Cuba as *lucumi*) is an amalgam of the Yoruba religion of West Africa and Roman Catholicism. It appeared in Cuba during the seventeenth century after slaves from Africa were brought to the island to cultivate and harvest sugarcane and other crops grown by Spanish settlers. In contrast to Catholicism, Santería is polytheistic. A number of deities, known as *orishas*, were originally worshiped in Africa, but over time, as missionaries brought Catholicism to Africa and the Caribbean, they became the rough equivalent of Catholic saints in Santería doctrine.

"Santería is a curious mixture of the magic rites of the Yorubas and the traditions of the Catholic Church," says anthropologist Migene González-Wippler in her book *Santería: African Magic in Latin America*, one of the key works on the subject, written after her experiences with its adherents in New York. "All the legends and the historical arguments that surround the lives of Jesus, Mary, and the Catholic saints are of great importance to the *santero*."

But Santería is also mostly primitive magic, González-Wippler adds. "Its roots are deeply buried in the heart of Africa."

The accoutrements of Santería are very much in evidence at Mora's *botánica*, as they are in other *botánicas* around the city. For a start, the beautifully crafted statue of Saint Barbara in the store window, though representative of the pantheon of Catholic saints, is also symbolic of the Santería *orisha* known as Chango, the deity believed to have power over lightning and fire. That symbolic connection appears to stem from the legend that at the moment she was killed, Saint Barbara's executioner was struck down by a bolt of lightning. By the herbal display case hang colored beaded necklaces, known as *collares*, which are used in the early part of the process of initiation of a person to the rank of *santero*. Made under elaborate ceremonial rules, the necklaces have the effect of lending a person powers needed for protection until he or she develops the right relationship with the deities, according to Garrison.

Hanging from other shelves in Botánica Santa Barbara are strings of seashells. While at first glance they might look like tourist souvenirs, the shells, known as *caracoles*, are said to be highly prized items for the *santero*. Known as a *diloggun* when they are strung together, the shells are used as ways of talking with the saints. The shells are thrown or allowed to fall onto a table or other surface, and their arrangement indicates a message that is read by a *santero*.

To become a *santero* requires going through a number of rituals and ceremonies, with final initiation by a *babalawo* (godfather) or *santera* (godmother), according to González-Wippler. Once a person is made a *santero*, he or she is invested with the power to give consultations in the community, a status that holds a great deal of power and prestige. People who are sick, gamblers in desperate straits, lovers who have been jilted, wives and husbands who suspect their spouses are having affairs, people seeking success in careers, or those facing some ill-defined anxiety—all consult the *santero* to solve their problems. People can invest hundreds and even thousands of dollars in items used to cast spells. If the spells seem to work, the practitioner can grow wealthy.

"Highly successful *santeros* become rich very rapidly," said González-Wippler. "They own real estate and profitable businesses, and have staggering bank accounts."

Magic is an element intrinsic to Santería, and because the belief system views nature as the source of power, something natural seems to be needed for the spells to work. "The most basic spell in Santería will require a plant, an herb, a stone, a flower, a fruit, or an animal," says González-Wippler. It is with those elements that any *santero*, she writes, is believed to be able to cure a "simple headache or a malignant tumor." While there is no way to test such a claim, it does appear that Santería relies on a number of medicinal plants that, when used together in a ritual inititation drink known as the *omiero*, may be viewed as an elixir. Gonzalez-Wippler lists twenty-one herbs she was told are used in the sacred drink. Four of them, as noted elsewhere in this book, are used widely in Hispanic cultures as medicinal plants: basil, sarsaparilla, mint, and aniseed. Other plants used in the mix, such as lettuce, watercress, river fern, and vervain, are consumed as food. True, the *omiero* is not used in Santería as a medicine. But for the Hispanic cultures that value magical and spiritual powers, the use of the medicinal herbs in the rituals appears to reinforce and validate the traditional uses of such plants for health care practices, even if it is done outside the bounds of Santería.

At one time, health officials expressed concern about the availability in *botánicas* of mercury under the name *azogue*, a substance imbued with significance in *espiritismo*, Santería, and voodoo. A person would carry a small amount of it in a leather pouch or sprinkle it at home or in an automobile for good luck or to ward off evil spirits and bad energy. Sometimes it was burned or used in baths. The problem is that mercury can harm the nervous system, particularly in children and developing fetuses. The sale of *azogue* was once commonplace; a study done by Drs. Luis Zayas and Philip O. Ozuah and published in the *American Journal of Health* found that nearly 93 percent of the New York *botánicas* polled in 1995 sold mercury. But a public education campaign by health officials appeared to have stemmed its sale in *botánicas*, according to one city official.

Somewhere in between the world of *espiritismo* and Santería is the role of the *curandero*, the lay curer in Hispanic communities who tries to heal a person's soul and body together in the practice known as *curanderismo*. Like Santería, *curanderismo* has African roots. Some of the spiritual beliefs and medical practices of black slaves brought to Mexico found their way into this form of Hispanic folk medicine, according to Elena Avila. The Spanish influence, Avila says, came with the belief that the responsibility for sickness was intertwined with curses, magic, and sin.

"In general, illness was considered an effect of a possession by evil spirits, resulting from not following God's laws," Avila writes. In her view, *curanderismo* evolved as a way for the indigenous cultures of Latin America to heal their loss of soul, known as *susto*, that resulted from the Spanish conquest of the Americas and the destruction of the local cultures.

In the Hispanic folk cultures, there is a standard list of diseases, both physical and emotional, that are treated by *curanderismo*. Some experts have likened the folk illnesses to the ancient Greek concept of imbalances in the four humors. Hispanics believe that a disorder of hot and cold principles causes the problems afflicting a patient. Under this belief system, stomach problems can occur if cold food or drink is ingested continually, causing contractions and spasms that can lead to indigestion, diarrhea, and other gastric upsets. Diseases are characterized as either "hot" or "cold," signifying an imbalance that has to be addressed by remedies that restore the equilibrium in the body through the use of a hot or cold therapy. For instance, a respiratory condition such as asthma may be considered a "cold" illness that is best treated by keeping warm.

While the hot-and-cold principle of diseases helps

explain the logic and method of treatment used for some folk illnesses, understanding the illnesses requires a brief look at their classic descriptions. The physical ones are *empacho*, *bilis*, and *mal aire*, while the mental or emotional illnesses are *mal ojo*, *mala suerte*, and *susto*.

Empacho is defined as a blockage of the stomach or gastrointestinal tract caused by overeating or by ingestion of the wrong kind of food or a hard-to-digest food. This condition, which one survey found that 64 percent of Hispanics polled reported suffering from at some point, leads to vomiting, constipation, or diarrhea. *Bilis* is rage, which Avila says is thought to be caused by excessive secretion of bile brought about by a person's chronic state of anger. *Mal aire*, which translates to "bad air," refers to exposure to night air that is believed to cause colds and earaches, a belief that Avila says is based on an old Aztec concept that there are particles in the air that can make a person sick.

The emotional illnesses in Hispanic cultures are often defined in terms of transmission of energy between people, explanations that for some may border on the magical. *Mal ojo* has been referred to as a belief that illness in a child may result from a person with a "strong eye" merely looking at a child. It can come from too much attention being paid to the young one. *Mala suerte* is bad luck and is really an explanation of the emotional state of a person suffering from low self-esteem and despair who finds him- or herself in a spiral of misfortune. *Susto* can come from some startling and traumatic event, which can cause insomnia, depression, and anxiety. There are also conditions resulting from curses and ghosts.

To heal the body and soul, *curanderos* use a variety of methods, from counseling to massage to herbal therapy.

But when it is apparent that a person's illness is beyond the ability of folk medicine, a good *curandero* will refer the patient to a conventional medical practitioner. According to Avila, a majority of *curanderos* use herbs in their work, as do other ethnic healers. This is another way in which medicinal plants have become an essential part of Hispanic folk medicine. The plants may be used by *curanderos* as treatment for a specific illness or in one of a number of cleansing rituals known as *limpias*.

Within the folk medical traditions of Hispanics, the lines of demarcation between the various practices are never rigid. There is frequently a crossover of rituals and practices. *Curanderismo's* principle of mending the soul and the body as a unit, *espiritismo's* belief in a world of spirits paralleling the material one, and the magical practices of Santería are all often closely intertwined. A *curandero* may practice *espiritismo*, and a spiritist or medium may also practice Santería. Some *curanderos* are also reputed to dabble in black witchcraft or *brujería*. Whatever the practice, medicinal plants play an important role.

To be sure, each approach is different, but all incorporate concepts that are beyond the bounds of the more "rational" Western medicine. It is the reliance on the spiritual and the magical that is important for anyone attempting to understand alternative medical practices or wanting to act as a health care professional within an ethnic community. This does not mean that there has to be a wholesale acceptance of the belief system underlying the practices. But some medical experts believe a doctor-patient relationship is better served by an atmosphere of trust and understanding than by one in which a trusted folk remedy is seen as bizarre or worthless. But while it may be important to understand and tolerate the melding of the spiritual and the medical that goes on in the Hispanic communities, it is also crucial to realize that sometimes the traditional healing systems can be dangerous.

Just how dangerous reliance on traditional healing methods can be is demonstrated by some cases that have made their way into the medical journals. Two cases in particular involve the practices of particular *curanderos* active among ethnic Mexicans; one instance took place in Texas and another in Mexico. Both cases involved children, and in each incident the child died.

In the Texas case, a twelve-year-old Mexican-American girl had been feeling ill for several months, exhibiting nausea and lack of appetite. Her grandmother was a noted *curandera* in the city where the family lived, and not surprisingly the old woman's advice was sought in an effort to help the child. The child, the grandmother surmised, was suffering from *empacho*, a blocked gastrointestinal tract, and cups of chamomile tea were prescribed, no doubt with the strong expectation that the little girl would get better.

But the child did not improve and in fact remained sick for months. A regular doctor diagnosed the condition as anemia and implored the family to allow further laboratory work—a request that was denied. Lesions and bruises appeared on the little girl's body, and her condition markedly deteriorated. A priest gave the last rites of the Roman Catholic Church, and an ambulance finally took the child to a hospital. It was there that doctors discovered the girl was suffering from leukemia. She died within five hours of being admitted.

The details of this case were first published by Wallace

W. Marsh, M.D., and Mary Eberle, M.D., in an article in the February 1987 issue of the journal *Texas Medicine*. According to Marsh and Eberle, the actions of the family were dictated by a number of Hispanic cultural beliefs about health and health care. For instance, there is the belief that a good doctor would know the right diagnosis on the first visit. As a result, the authors say, "the family was more likely to accept the *curandera* grandmother's immediate diagnosis of *empacho* rather than the judgement of the physician who had requested further tests." Blood drawing in particular, according to Marsh and Eberle, is frowned on in the culture, which also views hospitals as hostile places where a person goes only to die.

Another case illustrates how some folk healers may recklessly apply traditional medicines, also with tragic results. Such was the case of another Mexican child, one not quite three years old, who was treated by a local *curandera* in Mexico, presumably for a gastrointestinal problem such as worms or diarrhea. The healer administered oil of epazote *(Chenopodium graveolens)*, also known as wormseed. In Latin cultures, epazote is a traditional remedy for intestinal parasites and intestinal gas, and sometimes is used as a sedative. The plant oil known as ascaridol, which is effective against intestinal parasites, is said to be the major component of oil of epazote.

However, the dose administered by the *curandera*, according to a report of the case published in a Mexican medical journal, amounted to 1,560 milligrams of ascaridol, twenty-six times higher than the recommended dose for such a young child and well above the 1,000-milligram dose reported as lethal for humans. The child went into a coma, suffered seizures and other problems, and died. An autopsy revealed swelling of the brain, pancreatitis, and other problems.

A review of medical literature has not shown further recurrence of incidents like the Texas leukemia case or the epazote poisoning. That would indicate that either the cases go unreported or the vast majority of *curanderos* refer patients who appear to have serious physical illnesses to professional medical personnel for further treatment, as Elena Avila has stated.

In his shop on Broadway, surrounded by his herbs, incenses, magic sprays, prayer candles, and Santería artifacts, Antonio Mora personifies the special commerce that has evolved in Hispanic communities to supply the unique blend of spiritual and health practices that are so important to the immigrant cultures. But it is Lisa, the woman who acted to protect the store, who symbolizes the bridge between the spirit world and that of the flesh. No one is certain about the number of adherents to Santería or how many people are curious about the religion. But it is clear from a look around Mora's store that there is interest at all levels of society. The musician Tito Puente used to visit the *botánica*—Mora showed me photographs of one of Puente's visits to the store the year before the famous bandleader died. And high up on a shelf is a picture of Yankee pitcher Orlando "El Duque" Hernández.

In her last act of protection against what she believed to be evil energy, Lisa waved a maraca in the sign of the cross, first with slow rattles and then faster, all the while backing up as she faced the inside of the *botánica* door. Satisfied she need not do anything else, Lisa sat down and fixed me in her gaze. Through Mora she explained that at the age of thirteen in the Dominican Republic she started working as a medium.

"She was born with this," Mora said about her gift.

Lisa was sitting back in her chair, looking serene and content, a knowing smile on her face as she glanced out onto Broadway.

CHAPTER TWO

The Herbal Tradition

Some 2,500 miles away from Botánica Santa Barbara, in the city of San José, the capital of Costa Rica, is another kind of marketplace. The Mercado Central, as its name implies, is the focal point of commerce in this Central American city. It is a tired, painted building on the main concourse in town, the Avenida Central, three blocks from the city's main square. The place is old and shows it. Inside the main passageway of the market is a stale smell, a commingling of the odors of old cardboard boxes, wet wood, fried rice, and animal fat. With the shops and stalls lined up along narrow alleyways, the market resembles a Middle Eastern bazaar. The floor is worn maroon tile over concrete, all with the accumulated grime from years, maybe decades, of feet of passing Ticas, as native Costa Ricans call themselves. A sheet metal roof is punctuated with an occasional skylight.

Since the market is enclosed, there is a constant drone that resembles that heard in New York's Grand Central Terminal. A waitress, looking bored and moving slowly among the tables of a marketplace restaurant, tries to entice passersby to stop.

"What will you have?" she said in Spanish over and over to no one in particular. "What will you have?"

Not far from the main entrance, down one of the alleyways, is Alfredo's business. He did not reveal his last name but had no problem talking about his livelihood. His job in San José is similar to that of Antonio Mora's in New York, selling medicinal herbs.

Alfredo's store is really just an open market stall without walls, known to the merchants as a *tramo*. It is covered with so many plants that it looks like a hut from the South Sea islands. Stems of aloe vera hang from the walls, looking with their serrated edges like trophies from a swordfish. Fresh flowering chamomile, its fragrant smell easily masking the odor of the marketplace, is stuffed into pails of water. Eucalyptus, with its own menthol-like aroma, adds to the scent that permeates the surroundings. Other plants are piled high along the shelves, some dry, some fresh. Stacks of bark from the cinchona tree, the source of quinine, used to fight malaria, sit next to chunks of sarsaparilla, which is used as a health tonic, and mozote, which is believed to help stomach ulcers.

Alfredo works six days a week at the business, one of about a half dozen competing *tramos de hierbas* in the market. One of twelve brothers in his family, the thirty-eight-year-old Alfredo has known only the way of life of the *tramo*, as did his father. Those who sell medicinal plants in Costa Rica tend to come from long lines of entrepreneurs who have carved out a family niche.

A few turns down another alley in the market is the *tramo* run by Carlos and Eugenia Asturias. Eugenia, who works as a schoolteacher, said that their business, Tramo de Hierbas Margarita, was passed down from Carlos's grandmother to his mother and, as far as anybody can remember, has always been in the Mercado Central. They have a product that is much in demand.

In a country that seems blessed with an eternally spring-like climate, Costa Rican herbal merchants such as Alfredo and the Asturias family have a large, seemingly never-ending source of supply. What they do not grow themselves they buy from any number of itinerant herb and plant gath-erers, men and women who round up bushels of plant ma-terial from the lush tropical rain forests and fertile plains that comprise so much of the countryside surrounding the capital city. Tying their products into large white bags, the herb gatherers make their way to San José's central market, where buyers await them.

Experts in Costa Rica say that the reliance of the popula-tion here on medicinal plants is strong, as it is in many Latin American countries. Part of the reason for that is the cost of medical care in a country where money is not plenti-ful. Some who monitor Central American economies say expensive drugs produced by the large pharmaceutical companies are scarce.

"Medical services are really expensive," explains Victor, who runs the fish counter next to Alfredo's herb stand, "so many more poor people do this." He gestures at the rich va-riety of medicinal plants piled around the stall.

Victor maintains that herbal remedies have always been used in Costa Rica and that they are more appealing now because medical care is so costly. Victor does not know if the plants are as effective as Western medicines. But as persuasive and correct as the economic argument might be for their use, the tradition of using medicinal plants is one that is deeply intertwined with the cultures of Latin America.

The ancient Maya, Aztec, and Inca cultures had devel-oped their own sophisticated systems for using medicinal plants before the Spanish Conquest in the early part of the sixteenth century. These three Indian cultures were centered in three distinct areas. Mayans occupied what is now Guatemala, Belize, southern Mexico, Honduras, and the northern part of Costa Rica. The Incas had an empire that included a wide swath of territory stretching from Peru into what is now western Argentina and northern Chile. The empire of the Aztecs centered on an area where Mexico City stands today.

Though there is not a great deal of written material from those civilizations to rely on, historians agree that herbal medicines were an established part of the health systems in those societies. The Aztecs in particular are believed to have had a pharmacopoeia of about 1,500 medicinal plants. Historians say that botanical gardens flourished throughout the empire. The written record kept by the Aztecs of their history and culture was largely destroyed by the Spanish after Cortés arrived in 1519. But around 1570, King Philip II of Spain sent Francisco Hernández, a court physician, to Mexico to investigate medicinal plants and general medical practices in the area. The work took over seven years and what was for that time a substantial amount of money. Hernández died before his task was completed and a large part of his compilation was destroyed in a fire, although a copy with information on 1,200 herbs and plants survived and was ultimately rediscovered in Europe. A similar medical text done earlier by Martín de la Cruz, a Christianized Aztec, also survived.

It was a Spaniard who was responsible for one of the most ambitious written works on the Aztecs. Father Bernardino de Sahagún learned the Náhuatl language and, with help from Aztec nobles and scribes, wrote *A General*

History of the Affairs of New Spain, which was a comprehensive look at much of the life in the newly conquered lands, including a large section on herbs and medicinal plants.

Mayan books did not fare well. Most were destroyed by the Spanish after the Conquest, with all that remains amounting to three codices written on bark paper, now housed in Europe. However, historians say that Mayan manuscripts from the seventeenth century listed many illnesses and the appropriate cures. Yucatán, where the Maya lived, had a large assortment of medicinal plants.

The Inca tradition of medicine was memorialized in an account written by Felipe Guamán Poma de Ayala, the offspring of a noble Peruvian family. In the fifteenth century he prepared a codex, *Prima Nueva Curonica*, that describes the medical practices and beliefs of the Incas. According to medical historian Helmut M. Boettcher, the codex described numerous plants, including species that have medicinal uses.

Historians agree that the ancient Indian cultures' medical traditions were tightly bound with elements of religion. The traditions survived, despite attempts at suppression, and though the Spanish did construct hospitals in the conquered areas, it appears that the Indians continued to rely mostly on their own traditional healers and medicinal plants for treatment.

Many of the healing plants familiar to Indians in one area of the Americas also grew in other areas. So as geographically separate as those three civilizations may have been, there was nothing to keep indigenous peoples throughout Latin America from sharing knowledge of plant pharmacology. It was also not long before European settlers and traders came to realize the benefits the New World botanicals could provide. Europe had been battered by virulent outbreaks of diseases such as the plague and syphilis, and the Americas, particularly the Caribbean, were looked to for new cures. In 1578, Nicholas Monardes of Seville wrote in his *Joyful Newes out of the Newe Founde Worlde* about a number of plant cures from the West Indies, such as China root and sarsaparilla, that were used as syphilis remedies. His interest sparked widespread interest in New World botanicals.

"Virtually all of the new plants and drugs that excited the medical world of the sixteenth and seventeenth centuries were exotics," Barbara Griggs writes in her history of plant medicine, *Green Pharmacy*. "From 1602 when England at last signed a peace treaty with Spain, imports of the plants from the Spanish colonies had increased by leaps and bounds."

According to Griggs, about 70 percent of the plant stocks of the European apothecaries were imported from either the Far East or the Americas, including medicinals such as sarsaparilla, balsam of Tolu, balsam of Peru, and sassafras. Writing and compiling material in the sixteenth century, the Spanish prelate Sahagún also reported about a variety of purges, diuretics, febrifuges, and sedatives the Aztecs used, including balsam of Tolu, sarsaparilla, and valerian.

One of the biggest botanical discoveries during the post-Conquest period in the New World was the bark of the cinchona tree, which had for years been used by the Indians of Peru and Ecuador to treat malaria, a disease that had ravaged parts of the Mediterranean. The legend sometimes repeated in historical accounts is that a Spanish soldier sick with malaria drank from a pool of water into which a cinchona tree had fallen. Chemicals of the tree bark had seeped into the water, which revived the ailing soldier. There are other legends about the discovery of the restorative powers of this special rain forest tree. But historians generally agree that it was a European missionary who in 1663 first reported the indigenous use of cinchona bark, telling his order about a tree growing in Peru "which they call the Fever tree in the country of Loxa, whose bark is the colour of cinnamon . . . it has produced miraculous cures in Lima." Eventually Jesuits shipped the bark back to Rome, where one cardinal, after being cured by the substance, ordered that every sample of the bark have a little leaflet with instructions on how to mix it in a glass of white wine in order to cure a fever, according to Griggs's historical account of that period. There was business intrigue over cinchona, too. One British apothecary, James Talbot, set himself up as a fever specialist who promoted his own cure over the use of cinchona. He gained wide renown and warned customers against using cinchona. But according to Griggs, after Talbot's death, in 1682, Louis XIV of France revealed that Talbot had in fact been using a mixture of rose leaves, lemon juice, wine, and an infusion of cinchona.

The flow of medicinal plants was not only from the New World to the Old. During the colonial period, a great many plants from Europe and the Middle East found their way to the Americas, where they were able to thrive in the hospitable climate and become a part of the local folk medicine practices. Chamomile, rue, and rosemary all became firmly planted in the herbal apothecaries of Latin America—as any visitor today to the herbal stalls in San José's Mercado Central can plainly see.

The herb stalls in San José, piled high with medicinal

plants, have the appearance of a cornucopia. The *tramos* cater to a market that very much believes in the efficacy of the folk remedies. But it is also a belief, it seems, that comes without a reliance on the spiritual and magical elements more prevalent farther north, in Mexico and the Caribbean. The herbs are used, Costa Ricans say, because people believe they work, not because of magic.

The lack of reliance on the spiritual elements in Costa Rica is illustrated by the way the herb merchants sell their wares. No religious symbols are evident, no towering figures of saints or deities. Instead, hand-printed on white sheets of paper with black and red ink are the names in Spanish or English of various maladies or organs the plants are believed to be useful for: *próstata* (prostate), *asma* (asthma), *impotencia* (impotence), *leche materna* (mother's milk), *nervios insomnio* (insomnia), and so on. Under each ailment are listed the names of effective medicinal plants and how they are to be used.

Botanists have noticed some interesting differences between the indigenous medicinal plants and Western-style drugs, something that is evident from a perusal of the market signs in the San José herbal stands. Balick and his colleague Paul Alan Cox have noted that indigenous plants are more often used for "gastrointestinal (GI) complaints, inflammation, skin ailments, and ob-gyn disorders, whereas Western drugs are most often used to treat disorders of the cardiovascular and nervous systems, neoplasms [i.e., cancer], and microbial ailments."

Why is there such a difference? The reasons are found within the lifestyles of the cultures. Cardiovascular illness, cancers, microbial infections, and nervous system problems are bigger killers in Western cultures, compared with the lifestyles of indigenous peoples, who tend not to live as long and see diarrhea, maternity problems, and inflammations as more serious, wrote Balick and Cox. In fact, other researchers have noted that it has not been unheard of for infant mortality in some Amazon tribes to reach an astonishing 30 percent, with more than half of the deaths among children under one year old attributed to diarrhea, dysentery, or respiratory infections. Balick and Cox have also noted that traditional cultures are likely to avoid plants containing toxic substances that, while perhaps useful against cancer and cardiovascular problems, have a narrow dosage window that requires sophistication in the way they are used.

This is illustrated as well by the shortlist of medicinal plants that, under Costa Rican law, can be sold for remedial purposes. Under the Costa Rican practice, the market *tramos* can sell the medicinal plants as vegetables in their natural state. But once they are sold in stores as extracts, powders, soaps, or pills, the harvesting and processing of the plants are supposed to be more tightly controlled. At least in theory, the plants have to be properly identified, their chemical components must be assayed, and their purity acceptable. In practice, however, Costa Ricans say it is difficult to ensure that all of the medicinal plants harvested meet the expectations.

It turns out that while Costa Ricans traditionally rely on scores of medicinal plants, only a handful are officially recognized as safe for documented health-related uses. The shortlist includes chamomile, thyme, sarsaparilla, and mint verbena. Even though such plants have numerous traditional medicinal uses, under the Costa Rican regulatory scheme they are recognized for use either as an intestinal antispasmodic or to help urination, the kinds of physical problems that Balick and Cox note are most often treated with plants by indigenous peoples.

This modest listing of documented plants in Costa Rica, despite a vast cultural experience in Central America with plant medicine, is typical of what has gone on elsewhere. Very often governments, world organizations, and regulators have moved more cautiously, though at different paces depending upon location, in recognizing plants for use as folk medicine.

Standing by any of the herbal stalls in the San José market provides a visitor with a view of some of the most widely used medicinal plants in Hispanic cultures, from the southwestern United States and Mexico to South America. In fact, the most commonly used plants among Mexicans and Costa Ricans are similar. Asked which remedies they use most often, Mexicans on both sides of the Rio Grande in cities in Texas and Mexico listed chamomile, aloe vera, rue, anise, mint, wormwood, orange tree leaves, sweet basil, oregano, garlic, and rosemary. All but orange tree leaves are available in the Costa Rican market. Some two thousand miles south, in a women's health clinic in Chile, chamomile, oregano, rue, and rosemary are the key ingredients of a number of remedies listed in a recipe book. Clearly, while there are regional variations, there exists a basic core knowledge of herbal medicines among the many Latin cultures that stems from both the ancient Indian and the European peoples.

A sense of how deeply entrenched the use of medicinal plants is within the cultures of Latin America can be determined from a number of recent studies, some ongoing. There are so many plant species in Latin America that it has been impossible so far for any one group of researchers to determine all of the medicinal plants available. But one study in particular, focusing on the Caribbean basin and Central America, had by 1999 identified and studied 109 plants used in traditional healing practices. The review, done by the organization Traditional Medicine in the Island (TRAMIL), surveyed rural populations to find out which plants were commonly used to treat illnesses (serious conditions such as cancer and AIDS were excluded). Next they reviewed the chemical composition of the individual species, identified potential dangers, and made recommendations on their use. The results are published in a Caribbean pharmacopoeia and are part of an overall strategy by TRAMIL to spread valuable knowledge about safe medicinal plants and encourage their cultivation in order to provide Central Americans and Caribbean islanders with an affordable alternative to Western-style drugs.

About one-tenth of the plants surveyed by TRAMIL are considered toxic and their usage is discouraged. But a majority of the plants are either still under investigation or are considered to be safe. Among the latter are a number of medicinal plants familiar to the Hispanic cultures and sold by the *hierbas* vendors throughout the region: chamomile, peppermint, eucalyptus, ginger, papaya, annatto, and others. It is the same core group of medicinal plant products found continually throughout the Latino world.

Were they to work at herbal stands outside of Costa Rica, merchants such as Alfredo and the Asturias family would undoubtedly feel comfortable knowing that their products would be in demand among the local populace. Still, the herb vendors of San José have been facing uncertainty about where they might be conducting business in the years to come. Rumors keep circulating in the Mercado Central that some developers are interested in razing the hundred-year-old structure and building a modern complex. Some of the merchants simply do not know what the rebuilding plan would mean for them or if they would be able to stay. But if the herb traders did move, the customers would undoubtedly seek them out.

CHAPTER THREE

New Uses for Old Medicine

Lisa Conte and Dr. Alan Snow have careers that originally stemmed from different disciplines. Conte was steeped in the world of corporate finance and venture capital, while Snow, trained in biology and medical science, earned a reputation as a researcher in the field of Alzheimer's disease. Though their backgrounds are different, both became important players in the development of two medicinal plants from the Latin American rain forests as important products to treat disease in the twenty-first century. Conte's efforts led to a product derived from the plant dragon's blood. Snow helped develop the use of a derivative from the vine cat's claw that is believed to help some Alzheimer's patients. Their stories show how moments of inspiration, corporate commitment, and scientific research are coming together to develop new drugs from older traditions of medicine.

It was mid-1988 and Conte, a Dartmouth College graduate and American businesswoman not yet thirty years old, found herself climbing Mount Kilimanjaro, Africa's tallest peak and one of the world's most famous mountains. The fabled writer Ernest Hemingway had made it the focus of his famous story "The Snows of Kilimanjaro." Over the generations the lure of the mountain has inspired many, some wrapped up in their own sense of adventure and others seeking a more spiritual connection, to climb its slopes.

But before the grandeur of the summit, there is the work of the climb. At a height of 19,340 feet, with a gradual ascent that could take two or three days, Kilimanjaro does not seem like a punishing trek. There are no dangerous precipices or ice fields. But the volcanic mountain massif, which consists of three craters, poses a number of challenges on the way to the top. Climbers experience the heat and the cold. Rain forest growth, known to some as the "vegetable bog," often heralds the arrival of altitude sickness, making some climbers nauseous, weak, and laboring for breath.

Local entrepreneurs saw that there was a market for an elixir that promised to help those experiencing altitude sickness, and so they set up makeshift stands in the jungle area along the Kilimanjaro route. They hawked bottles of what Conte remembered to be "green goop," plant extracts of unknown origin—possibly sage, which some climbers say locals use to cure indigestion. One of her hiking companions happened to feel the effects of altitude. Hoping for something that would help, Conte's friend took some of the viscous fluid.

Looking at the green drink, Conte's hiking companion turned to her and said, "You know, Lisa, you should really do something about that someday." She meant, of course, finding a treatment for altitude sickness and making a business out of it, perhaps from a vegetable concoction much like that being sold along the Kilimanjaro trail.

Lisa Conte never did find a cure for altitude sickness. But that moment in the jungle by the mountain refreshment stand got her thinking about how plants might hold the key to better human health. This intellectual curiosity about plants stayed with Conte for several months, but as a venture capitalist in California, she had enough other things to keep her busy.

Things changed rather suddenly when a copy of *Smithsonian* magazine landed on Conte's desk a day before her thirtieth birthday. Glancing through the periodical, Conte found an article that dealt with the destruction of the world's rain forests and how the loss of so many plant resources threatened to deny humanity the chance to use global botanical resources to better human health.

It was a moment of epiphany for Conte. Why not, she thought, use the knowledge acquired from thousands of years of human experience to find medicines that were safe, effective, and new? The next day, her birthday, Conte told her colleagues at Technology Funding, Inc., where she was a vice president, that she was going to quit to found a company that would work to develop pharmaceuticals from the botanical resources of the rain forests before any more of that precious global resource was lost to the rapacious crush of cultivation and the logging industry. Conte's friends at Technology Funding talked her out of walking straight out the door in what must have looked to them like an impulsive move. Instead, they convinced her to stay affiliated with the venture capital firm under a special arrangement that would allow her to return to her old desk if things did not work out.

After six months of investigating on her own and talking with some of the best-known ethnobotanists in the field, Conte started Shaman Pharmaceuticals, Inc., in 1990. The company's goal was to develop pharmaceutical products derived from tropical plant sources, many of which grow in Latin America and have a long history of being used by indigenous and Hispanic cultures as medicinal plants.

A number of pharmaceutical companies had developed some medicines from plants and plant-based substances. But Shaman (the name is derived from the word for a man or woman who treats illness by communicating with the spirit world) was structured around the idea that state-of-the-art technology and science could be combined with knowledge of traditional medicinal plants to, as Conte says, "play a part in staving off destruction of the world's tropical rain forests and in developing novel pharmaceuticals for unmet medical needs as well." It was a strategy that would tap into the knowledge of Hispanic folk medicinal practices, further legitimizing a system of folk medicine that had for so long been viewed by many Western minds as quaint, inferior, or unproven.

Using credit cards, Conte and her associates borrowed $40,000 for initial funding before they had a business plan to entice venture capitalists to start kicking in more money. Conte remembers there was skepticism about such a business, even though the world was awash with environmental concerns, particularly about the rain forests. But soon stock offerings pulled in more money, and by 1996 Shaman had raised over $85 million through a combination of stock sales and venture capital.

One of the first things Shaman did was to pick among the best minds in the area of ethnobotany and science technology to develop a plan to screen plants used by native healers in Latin America, Africa, and Southeast Asia. The theory was that while random screening of plants might hit upon some important medicinal substances, a more channeled investigative approach, using the knowledge of indigenous cultures, might fast-track the discovery process.

This presented the researchers with a huge task. Tropical America alone had an estimated one hundred thousand plant species. Factoring in tropical zones elsewhere in the world, the estimate of the universe of plants rose to five hundred thousand. Yet even by the late 1990s, only about 1 percent of the plants had been screened by scientists for possible medical use. To narrow the search, Shaman began to focus on plants that healers in South and Central America, as well as other tropical areas, used for particular ailments. Then, according to Conte, the company's scientific strategy team would evaluate the plants, giving a high priority to some of them for further testing and analysis. Such a focused approach, company officials hoped, would allow them to pay attention to medicinal plants with a history of safe usage.

The Amazon rain forest area, a veritable hothouse of traditional Hispanic remedies, was a natural place for Shaman to focus some of its efforts. The region has been the source of a number of medicines over the centuries. Cinchona, the natural source of quinine, was one of the first such medicinal plants exploited. Quinine was so important that during World War II a number of U.S. scientists and officials carried out a massive campaign in Ecuador and other parts of the region to harvest cinchona bark so that it could be processed to create enough quinine for the American war effort in the Pacific. Japanese control of parts of the Far East had effectively denied the United States and its allies access to the quinine industry there, and a new source had to be exploited.

Curare was another plant substance from the Amazon that, while dangerous, in small amounts proved useful as a muscle relaxant. The *Pilocarpus jaborandi* tree, known as a sweat inducer and diuretic to the Indians of the Amazon, yielded the alkaloid pilocarpine, which has proved useful in treating glaucoma. There was also *Catharanthus roseus*, or rosy periwinkle, which led to the discovery of treatments for leukemia and Hodgkin's disease.

Inspired by the groundbreaking work done over the decades, scientists and drug companies have been looking more closely at the plants of Latin America. It was a nascent industry by the time Shaman came on the scene, and the company decided to work closely with the local healers and shamans who hold the institutional memories of their peoples' medicinal practices.

Among the most well known of the programs aimed at developing promising leads for drugs from the rain forest have been those involving the New York Botanical Garden, which contracted with pharmaceutical companies such as Merck and Pfizer, as well as the National Cancer Institute, to prospect for plants that may hold out the possibility of proving useful. The botanical garden established a policy of splitting any royalties it receives from rain forest drug development with institutions it works with in those forested areas. Other companies have set up foundations aimed at benefiting indigenous communities should drugs be developed from plants from that area. In fact, the sharing of the benefits of drug development became a central part of Shaman's business philosophy. The company formed the

Healing Forest Conservancy, a nonprofit California corpo-
ration with the goal of taking donated funds from product
profits to provide help to indigenous people in the countries
where Shaman went prospecting for useful plants. The conservancy is also focused on conserving traditional medicinal plants.

One of the first Shaman officials to go out into the field in
the search for new drugs was Steven R. King. After living for
about two years in Peru in the late 1970s, King had climbed
up the career ladder in the sciences. He worked in 1988 as
a research associate for an arm of the National Academy of
Sciences. For five years prior to that he was a doctoral fel-
low at the New York Botanical Garden's Institute of Economic Botany, a unique and prestigious unit that carries
out research around the world into the economic relationship between people and plants. Just before he helped start
Shaman, King was the chief botanist for Latin America at
the Nature Conservancy in Arlington, Virginia.

Leading Shaman's scientific strategy team, King traveled
to the interior of Brazil and sought out healers he had once
known as well as others he would meet for the first time.
From colleagues back in the United States, King had heard
about dragon's blood, a medicinal plant known in Spanish
as sangre de drago and scientifically as *Croton lechleri*. A
tall rain forest tree that grows in the Amazon River basin,
dragon's blood is known for producing a gummy latex with
a deep reddish color, hence the popular name. The resin of
related species of trees had a history of being used in varnishes. But one species of the latex-bearing tree grown in
the northwest Amazon also had a widely known history of
use as a medicine. In fact, says King, the resin was used in
South America for coughs, as a topical application for

wounds, and to treat diarrhea and other gastrointestinal problems. It also had proved useful in healing surgical wounds. The tree was generally not cut down to harvest the resin; rather, its bark was scored to allow the fluid to escape.

According to researchers who have studied dragon's blood, the latex was sold in Central America and in Andean countries under at least twenty brand names. "These manufacturers sell small quantities of the liquid in bottles for hepatitis, diabetes, ulcers, cancer prevention, tonsillitis, as an anti-inflammatory, and to enhance fertility and weight loss" as well as for use as a vaginal wash and treatment for hemorrhoids and acne, according to an article published in the scientific journal *Phytomedicine*. Clearly, dragon's blood had a significant place in the world of Latin American folk medicine, especially as a remedy for cold and flu symptoms, says Conte. The question was whether it held the promise for development into a pharmaceutical product.

Respiratory syncytial virus (RSV) is a common problem, particularly among young children. The virus causes flulike symptoms and accounts for numerous hospitalizations. Taking some dragon's blood samples back to the United States, King and his colleagues screened resin extracts in an effort to see what effect it might have on RSV and other viruses, including those responsible for various forms of influenza, herpes, and hepatitis. At that time, only one plant-derived substance was being used as an antiviral medicine, so the discovery of another such compound would have an impact.

The initial lab tests with animals did not uncover any significant toxicity in dragon's blood. In terms of antiviral activity, the dragon's blood derivative, known as SP-303,

was found to exhibit potent activity against cell cultures of
RSV, influenza A, and parainfluenza virus, according to a
report published in *Phytomedicine*. The SP-303 derivative
was also shown to have antiviral activity against two types
of herpes viruses that had been resistant to some commercial preparations already on the market, as well as against
two types of hepatitis viruses. The results were encouraging, and King and his colleagues at Shaman decided to apply to the Food and Drug Administration for permission to
conduct clinical trials in humans in an effort to develop a
drug to combat RSV.

Generally, the FDA drug development process involves
three stages of clinical study, all of which have to be successfully navigated before a product can be approved for
general use. The initial trials, known as phase I, involved
screening SP-303 in about 120 adults who received varying
doses. The test results, according to Conte in a report she
later published, indicated that the drug had no significant
adverse effects in adults. A follow-up study in the spring of
1993 among children infected with RSV also indicated that
SP-303 was safe. No doubt buoyed by the phase I test results, in early 1994 Shaman embarked on phase II trials to
determine, among other things, more about the drug's
safety and its pharmacokinetics, or the way it is absorbed,
metabolized, and eliminated by the human body. It was at
the phase II level, according to Steven King, that things
started to get bumpy.

In an interview, King said that the FDA looked over the
results of the phase II trials and said that SP-303 was not
bioavailable; in other words, it could not be found in the
blood of people who had taken it. In such a case, it is difficult to explain how it could act on, say, the lungs, King

noted. The agency did not want to proceed with the study, and at that point Shaman's attempt to develop a drug to combat RSV in children had hit a roadblock.

But as one door closed, another seemed to open. Dragon's blood was widely known in Latin America to be useful for treating gastrointestinal problems, particularly diarrhea. The plant substance treated diarrhea by inhibiting the secretion of water into the intestines, which causes loose and watery stools. Diarrhea was a common health problem, frequently inconveniencing travelers, particularly in the tropics. Some twenty-six million antidiarrhea prescriptions are written worldwide each year to treat traveler's diarrhea alone, according to some estimates. But it had become a scourge for patients with AIDS, who could be racked by debilitating attacks for weeks at a time. While discouraging development of SP-303 as a drug for RSV, the federal agency encouraged Shaman to try to use it for the development of a treatment for diarrhea.

In 1996 Shaman, with the cooperation of an expert in travel medicine at the University of Texas Medical Center at Houston and Baylor College of Medicine, began a phase II study of SP-303 in the treatment of traveler's and nonspecific diarrhea. The results were encouraging. Of some seventy-five patients treated with acute diarrhea, including the traveler's syndrome, almost 90 percent experienced a rapid return to normal bowel function after taking the drug, according to results released by Shaman in November 1996. There were no significant adverse reactions and most patients had no recurrence, according to the study. SP-303 was rechristened with the name Provir.

Shaman announced it was planning to expand the phase II study to hundreds more patients and in 1997 expanded the trial again to include diarrhea in AIDS patients. The test results, released in July 1998, continued to be positive. One part of the trials showed Provir was effective among a sample of Americans traveling to Jamaica and Mexico, while a second part showed that the drug was helpful in clearing up diarrhea among Venezuelan nationals with acute watery diarrhea. Another aspect of the study involved fifty-one AIDS patients at two hospitals in California, who also seemed to do well. Test results published in October 1997 showed that those treated with Provir experienced a drop in the frequency of bowel movements and the weight of their stools.

With the Provir AIDS test results so encouraging, in 1998 Shaman received a "fast-track" designation from the FDA that would allow it to expedite development of the drug for AIDS-related diarrhea. If all went well, an application for approval to market a pharmaceutical product could move quickly. Dragon's blood held out the promise of help to AIDS patients, and Shaman was close to fulfilling one of its key goals: to develop novel human pharmaceutical products from tropical plants used in folk medicine.

But then problems arose when some FDA-approved drugs began to prove troublesome and dangerous once they became available to the public, despite the fact they had gone through the agency drug approval process. Two products proved to be too risky. Apparently concerned about such dangerous developments, the FDA wanted to slow down some of its fast-track programs, including the one involving Provir.

"So the FDA kind of backtracked and wanted to go by the book and not fast-track [Provir]," King recalled. The agency, he said, wanted to see "a little more data" and asked for another clinical trial.

"That popped us," remembered King. The company had already spent millions on the earlier trials and developing Provir. With no product line on the market and debt already high, Shaman was in no position to raise the millions of dollars needed for the further studies being asked for by the FDA. Provir, and by extension dragon's blood, were unlikely to turn into pharmaceutical products in the United States.

Shaman's filings with the Securities and Exchange Commission showed that it had incurred significant losses each year since the company was founded in 1989. As of mid-1999 the company had not generated any product sales, since its efforts had been devoted to developing drugs from traditional plants, according to SEC filings. Crippled in its attempt to launch Provir as a drug and with virtually no cash on hand, Shaman in late 1998 decided on some dramatic moves. The company closed down its pharmaceutical development operation and fired about 65 percent of its workforce. Shaman also tore up its old business model, based on developing pharmaceutical products, and decided to restructure and focus instead on the development and marketing of dietary supplements.

If Shaman was going to stay alive and not walk away from a decade of developing products from plants and a database of over 2,600 tropical plants, the dietary supplement business made a lot of sense. Not only was that market large in the United States—it was estimated to be at least $12 billion a year in sales in 1997, of which $4 billion was of botanical products—there was every indication that it would grow, particularly as the health-conscious baby boomer population began to age and plant products found a growing acceptance.

As part of the 1999 restructuring, Shaman in the fall of
that year began marketing the product SB-Normal Stool
Formula as a dietary supplement on the Internet and
through mail order and telephone sales, as well as in certain stores. This was the consumer version of the product
once known as Provir, and while the new name might not
have sounded as snappy, it could be very useful for persons
suffering from AIDS-related diarrhea.

Shaman was able to change direction as quickly as it did
because the marketing of a plant product as a dietary supplement is much easier than marketing it as a pharmaceutical. No expensive and lengthy trials are required, and
under the federal Dietary Supplement Health and Education Act of 1994, dietary supplements are not subject to
FDA premarket approval. That does not mean that the supplements are allowed to be marketed without regulation.
Manufacturers are not allowed to tout them as cures or
remedies for any specific ailment or condition. Instead, a
dietary supplement can bear a label saying it promotes or
maintains a certain bodily function, such as prostate health
in men or normal stool formation. The supplements also
are subject to quality control standards and cannot be mis-
labeled or adulterated.

Shaman also was exploring in late 1999 the marketing of
a number of other botanical products in addition to the
stool formula. One of them was Virend, another derivative
of dragon's blood that was useful against the herpes virus.
Herpes is a chronic and sometimes debilitating sexually
transmitted disease, and earlier tests with dragon's blood
extracts showed that the botanical substance was toxic to
the virus causing the disease. No longer able to spend millions of dollars on lengthy clinical trials, Shaman mulled

licensing Virend as a cosmetic cream for oral and genital herpes, said a company official. In filings with the SEC, Shaman said it was also planning to develop a diet system aimed at disorders related to diabetes. In addition, the company was working on products dealing with gastrointestinal relief, sleeping aids, calming agents, and products for weight management.

By mid-2000 Shaman, with nearly eight months' experience in marketing the stool formula, decided to expand its efforts. The company announced in May 2000 that it would enlarge its marketing and sales efforts to target more parts of the consumer diarrhea market. This was meant to include people who had irritable bowel syndrome, were undergoing chemotherapy and radiation treatments, had had bone marrow or organ transplantation procedures, or were experiencing the side effects of medication. Shaman also announced that it was cutting the price of its SB-Normal Stool Formula.

Unlike the scientists and executives at Shaman, Alan Snow was not into this herbal stuff. None of the dietary supplement crazes that had come into and out of fashion in the United States had had much appeal to him. As a man of science, dealing with the real and verifiable, it is hard to imagine that Snow would give much of a thought to the products on health food store shelves, much less a market stall selling herbal remedies, as a way of bettering his body and spirit.

A Canadian by birth, Snow obtained his Ph.D. in 1986 from Queen's University in Kingston, Ontario, and moved on to the University of Washington in Seattle, where he began to delve into his specialty, an area of biochemistry that

deals with the dynamics of a particular kind of cellular dis-
ruption affecting the human brain and leading to Alzheimer's
disease. Alzheimer's afflicts an estimated twelve million
elderly people worldwide, including about four million in
the United States, robbing them of their memory and other
mental faculties. Alzheimer's is seen as a long-range problem for Americans as the nation's baby boomer population
ages.

It was fortuitous that Snow came across one of the most
promising uses of a derivative of cat's claw, a traditional
Hispanic medicinal plant. Seeking the source of substances
that might be useful in creating a drug to fight Alzheimer's,
Snow and his colleagues looked at the shelves of a local
health food store in Seattle for an idea. They came across a
bottle of capsules of cat's claw, or una de gato. "It was just
lying around," said Snow in an interview.

Known botanically as *Uncaria tomentosa*, cat's claw is
widely used in Latin America and has found its way into
the American market. A woody vine with sharp thorns at
the base of its leaves—hence its popular name—cat's claw
grows throughout South and Central America in elevated
areas. It has been used traditionally for over two thousand
years by Peruvian Indians and has been used to stimulate
the immune system, as an anti-inflammatory for arthritis, to
treat wounds, and for cancer. It is sold in market stalls in
South and Central America as cut wood, in capsules, and
in tea bags; in the United States it is available through
botánicas, health food stores, and supermarkets as a bark
powder.

What drew Snow and his colleagues to take a closer look
at cat's claw was the fact that it contained a number of
plant substances that were found to protect the immune

system and body cells. For a start, says Snow, cat's claw contains flavonoids, which have the ability to protect human cells from oxidation. In addition, it contains a number of alkaloids that, he says, enhance the ability of certain of the body's white blood cells to attack invading organisms.

These and other attributes contained in the chemical makeup of cat's claw made the plant look promising for studies that had been on Snow's mind during a major project at his laboratory at the University of Washington. His work was aimed at determining what was responsible for causing Alzheimer's and researchers had focused attention on the persistence of beta-amyloid protein in the brain as a cause for the disease. Under the right conditions, the protein creates fibers, called amyloid fibrils, in the brain. These fibrils, tests showed, may be responsible for the kind of neurodegeneration observed in Alzheimer's patients. If they could find a way to interfere with the formation of the brain amyloid deposits, Snow and his colleagues believed, people who have Alzheimer's might be helped at both the early and late stages of the illness.

The interest in cat's claw was not the first time science had turned its attention to a medicinal plant in an effort to combat Alzheimer's. Human studies done with ginkgo biloba, a plant that has gained popularity as a memory-enhancing substance, showed that Alzheimer's patients who were given doses of ginkgo scored higher on memory tests compared with a group that took a placebo. Scientists believed the antioxidant properties of the plant might contribute to the effects seen in the studies.

Snow and his colleagues went about testing the cat's claw sample, making unique derivatives from it, as well as testing hundreds of other natural compounds, to see what could disrupt the formation of this brain plaque. Using laboratory rats as subjects, the researchers discovered that a derivative of cat's claw prevented the formation of amyloid deposits, and they reported those results at the Sixth International Conference on Alzheimer's Disease and Related Disorders in Amsterdam in July 1998. It was a breakthrough.

The extraction of the chemical from cat's claw was carried out by a company Snow cofounded named Proteo-Tech, a Washington State–based biotechnology firm. While the extraction process is a trade secret of the company, ProteoTech named the extract PTI-00703® and licensed its worldwide production and sale as a dietary supplement to Rexall Sundown of Florida. PTI-00703®'s antioxidant activity—a characteristic of a number of the constituent chemicals in cat's claw—is believed to help combat the debilitating and crippling effects of beta-amyloid fibrils in the human brain.

In April 1999, the results of in vivo rodent studies with the PTI-00703® compound were revealed at a conference in Washington, D.C. Around the same time, ProteoTech and Rexall began a pilot study with some mildly to moderately affected Alzheimer's patients. More clinical trials were launched as a prelude—if all went well—to approval by the FDA of PTI-00703® as a new dietary supplement for Alzheimer's. As of late 1999 there were only two such Alzheimer's medications on the market. The clinical trials were expected to last until early 2001.

If the effort does prove fruitful, it will be a major development in the world of pharmaceuticals. Interestingly, it was almost by chance that cat's claw found its way into the

Alzheimer's study, although researchers knew that any product that had antioxidant properties was a candidate for further investigation. Today Snow has a deep respect for the power that may be locked within plants used as folk medicines and which may make them useful in the fight against serious diseases. "Some of the most potent drugs on the market are derived from plants," he says. "Nature may have a lot of answers."

So two South American rain forest plants, each with a centuries-old role in Latin folk medicine, may hold the key to the treatment of some major health problems. But dragon's blood and cat's claw represent only an infinitesimal part of the plant life that could be examined for medical usefulness. At the National Cancer Institute, more than twelve thousand samples of plants collected from tropical areas are sitting in storage, just waiting to be studied by any pharmaceutical company willing to show interest and make the right commitment. Some of the flora was gathered by researchers at the New York Botanical Garden working in eight Latin American countries: Belize, Dominica, Dominican Republic, Ecuador, Guatemala, Guyana, Peru, and Trinidad. The aim of that collection effort was to gather plants with a history of use as traditional medicine in the hopes that they might one day be the source of important leads for future research.

Gordon M. Cragg, a National Cancer Institute official who works in the agency's natural products branch, part of its division of cancer treatment, is a firm believer in the ability of traditional plant medicines to continue their contribution to the health of people in many countries. He also thinks the prospects are good that pharmaceutical organizations will in the not-too-distant future agree to start testing plants in the National Cancer Institute plant repository—and that they will have good results, not only in the area of cancer and AIDS but also with tuberculosis, malaria, and heart disease.

"My feeling is in the next three to five years we will probably come up with some very exciting discoveries," said Cragg.

CHAPTER FOUR

Remedios

When the ancient Greek physician Dioscorides compiled his classic work on pharmacology, which dealt with more than six hundred plants and a thousand simple drugs, he called it *De materia medica*. In Latin that means "drugs." Over the centuries, the term *materia medica* has come to be synonymous with medical repertoires of all sorts, and so it could almost be used here. But since this book is about medicinal plants from the Hispanic cultures, the term *remedios* is the more apt title for this section, which provides detailed information about scores of the most widely used plant remedies within the various cultures of Latin America.

With a universe of plant life in tropical America that some botanists believe conservatively numbers over a hundred thousand species, there are hundreds of plants that are used in that part of the world for medicinal purposes. The aim of this book is to present description, facts, history, and medical knowledge for more than sixty of the most important species. Winnowing that list down from such a large universe proved to be a challenge. Aficionados may ask why a favorite plant—say, one that is popular in a particular area of Belize, Chile, or Mexico—was not included.

The question is a fair one. In one sense, the answer is very simple: Space allows only a certain number of the plants to be featured.

Still, a selection had to be made. In deciding which plants made the cut, a number of sources were consulted. Some medical journals actually listed common herbal and plant remedies used by Hispanics as a result of surveys done among immigrant populations around the United States. *Botánica* owners are also a good source of what plants are popular, as are herb vendors and farmers in Central America. Botanists, particularly those who travel to Latin America to gain firsthand knowledge of traditional medicines, and *curanderos*, who use plants in their healing practices, also have favorite remedies. Some plants, such as chamomile and aloe vera, are easy picks because they are so widely used by the general population. In other cases, as with jaborandi, which is not readily available to the public, its inclusion is based on the fact that one of its components, pilocarpine, has made a significant contribution to human medical knowledge. In the case of cinchona bark, it is easily purchased, but it is also blessed with a history that is especially interesting.

In the pages that follow, sixty-three key medicinal plants are discussed in depth, with nine descriptive entries for each species. After the Latin and common names are spelled out, each entry contains descriptive and historical information, mostly about the traditional medical uses for which the plants are noted. There is also information about the availability of the plant materials in the United States and, where available, about recommended dosages. Contraindications, medical precautions, and medical research information are also described.

Some of the headings in the sections about each plant are worth explaining in more detail because there are important caveats and background information that will give the reader a more complete understanding of some of the botanical and medical concepts involved.

Description: Physical characteristics of the plants, some quite unique, are detailed to give the reader a sense of how the plant looks in nature. The plants span the range from tall trees such as *Cinnamomum camphora*, the source of camphor, which reach heights of over a hundred feet in the jungles of the Amazon River basin, to herbs such as basil, which barely top a foot in height. Some produce fragrant flowers, while others are noted for more disagreeable aromas. A few, such as papaya, produce fruits that are staples, while other fruits have toxic seeds.

A number of botanical works were consulted to assemble the descriptions, but three publications in particular were useful as well in describing plant habitats. They are Julia F. Morton's *The Atlas of Medicinal Plants of Middle America: Bahamas to Yucatan*, James Duke's *CRC Handbook of Medicinal Herbs*, and Rosita Arvigo and Michael Balick's *Rainforest Remedies: One Hundred Healing Herbs of Belize*. These books and many more sources are listed in the bibliography. The Raintree Nutrition, Inc., Web site, maintained by author Leslie Taylor, was also helpful.

Traditional uses: These are compilations of medicinal uses made of the various plants in folk medicine practices over long periods of time, sometimes stretching back centuries to the times of the ancient Aztecs, Mayas, and Incas, as well as Romans, Greeks, Chinese, and Indo-Pakistanis. The list of traditional uses has been compiled from a review of published accounts, often derived from the experiences of healers, as well as a vast array of historical and botanical data. One Internet site that proved particularly helpful is that maintained by the United States Department of Agriculture. The agency's Ethnobotany Database, developed by Stephen M. Beckstrom-Steinberg, James A. Duke, and K. K. Wain, is accessible at the Internet address http://www.ars-grin.gov/duke/. The site consists of records on eighty thousand plants used around the world. Another Internet site that contains useful information about rain forest medicinal plants is one maintained by Raintree Nutrition, Inc., and Ms. Taylor. The site address is www.rain-tree.com.

At the end of this chapter and just before the descriptive listings, a list of maladies and medical conditions can be found. Along with each condition is listed an array of plants traditionally used to treat the illness. However, the reader should bear in mind that the listing of traditional medicinal uses of various plants in this book is not an endorsement of or recommendation for their use. Nor is any attempt made to diagnose any disease. It is said repeatedly in this book—and it is worth saying again—that a decision to use any botanical substance should be made only after consultation with a doctor.

Sometimes the traditional uses are described in medical terms. To keep the reader from having to reach for a medical dictionary, here is a short glossary of relevant terms that appear often:

1. *Abortifacient:* Substance that has the ability to induce an abortion
2. *Analgesic:* Substance that has the ability to reduce pain

3. *Antibacterial:* Substance that has the ability to cripple the growth of bacteria

4. *Anti-inflammatory:* Substance that has the ability to stop inflammation

5. *Antinociceptive:* Substance that has the ability to reduce sensitivity to painful stimuli or has an analgesic effect

6. *Astringent:* Substance that has the ability to constrict tissue or control bleeding

7. *Catarrh:* Condition of excessive secretions from an inflamed mucous membrane

8. *Cholalogue:* Substance that stimulates the flow of bile from the liver into the intestines

9. *Choleretic:* Substance that stimulates the liver to increase production of bile

10. *Demulcent:* Substance that soothes and stops irritation of mucous membranes

11. *Diuretic:* Substance that increases urinary flow

12. *Emmenagogue:* Substance that causes the onset of the menstrual period

13. *Expectorant:* Substance that loosens mucus in the throat or lungs

14. *Hypoglycemic:* Having to do with lowering blood sugar levels

15. *Laxative:* Substance that causes bowel movement

16. *Purgative:* Substance that has the ability to flush out the bowels

17. *Rheumatism:* Painful inflammation of muscle or joint

18. *Rubefacient:* Substance used to cause irritation to skin

19. *Stomachic:* Substance that promotes functional

activity of the stomach, improving appetite and digestion

Availability and dosage: In the United States, some of the plants listed in this book can be found in supermarkets or *botánicas* as fresh vegetables and fruit. Others can be found in powdered or capsule forms in health food stores. With the development of the Internet and the steady growth in the market for herbal substances, many of the botanical materials listed, particularly some of the products native to the Amazon area, can be purchased online.

As of late 1999, some of the online providers of botanical materials for traditional medicine include:

Rain-Tree.com:	http://www.rain-tree.com
Mothernature.com	http://www.mothernature.com
More.com:	http://www.more.com
Allherb.com:	http://www.allherb.com

Information about dosages for the medicinal plant substances varies widely depending on the herbalist consulted or the company marketing the product. For instance, one supplier recommends that the herb sarsaparilla be taken at a daily dosage of 2,490 mg in capsule form; another recommends 2,550 mg; a third recommends up to 9,000 mg daily. Liquid extracts of some herbs come with dosages expressed in numbers of drops. So, setting a dose is at best an inexact process and a course that is prudently navigated with the help of a physician or other qualified medical professional, with some attention paid to the manufacturer's label. Where there does not appear to be an established dosage, this book will note that dosages vary. It should also be kept in mind that growing conditions and climate may affect the chemical composition and medicinal qualities of a plant. The result is that different batches of the same herb may be of different quality. Quality control at the manufacturing level may also affect the final herbal product, and it is not unheard of for unscrupulous distributors to market a product as a particular herb when in fact it is not. Others may sell an adulterated product. This means that a consumer has to take the time to learn about the reliability of a distributor or manufacturer.

Traditional plant medicines and herbal remedies can be consumed in a number of ways, and the method of preparation will be dictated by the plant substance used. Herbal teas can be prepared from leaves or from pieces of bark, stem, or root. The process is relatively simple and involves steeping the materials in boiling or very hot water. Some herbal products are sold in convenient tea bag form. The listings in this book detail some ranges of doses found for teas in a review of herbal literature.

In addition, herbal substances, either in powdered form or extracts, are marketed in capsule form by a number of companies. They can be purchased by mail order or at health food stores. A few of the more well known ones, such as cat's claw or pau d'arco, can be purchased at supermarkets.

Other liquid forms in which herbal substances are consumed are called infusions, tinctures, or decoctions. *Infusions*, also made from dried herbs, are not tea, writes author Michael Castleman in his book *The Healing Herbs: The Ultimate Guide*. "Some herbalists use the terms interchangeably but the two are quite different," says Castleman. "Infusions are prepared like teas but they are steeped longer so they become considerably stronger." *Tinctures* are made by soaking a portion of the plant—which part depends on the particular traditional formula—in alcohol for up to two weeks. Often the plant parts are finely chopped, and the container is supposed to be shaken regularly. The resulting tincture is then used in solution or sometimes applied externally, depending on the medicinal plant. *Decoctions* are similar to infusions and are made by soaking crushed or finely chopped root, twig, or bark in boiling water and allowing it to simmer for up to twenty minutes. The mixture is then strained and the fluid is consumed by drinking.

Essential oils of some herbal plants are also available and are extracted by commercial distillation processes that are beyond the means of most consumers. However, a number of essential oils are available commercially from Internet or mail-order sites.

The Complete German Commission E Monograms: Therapeutic Guide to Herbal Medicines, which is published in the United States in collaboration with the American Botanical Council, lists recommended doses for many traditional herbal remedies, and they are sometimes referred to in this book. The commission is empowered by law to review herbal drugs and medicinal plants. The use of plants as medicine has been an accepted practice in Europe for many years (comprising an estimated 30 percent of all drugs sold in Germany, for instance), and the commission's collection of 380 monographs on herbal remedies is a logical outcome of such deep interest. The vast majority of the herbals are listed as approved, but a number are labeled as not approved, among them sarsaparilla. (One reviewer has cautioned that the work of Commission E is "not the final source" and notes that there is a lack of literature references and a failure to note possible fatal reactions to some plants.)

Contraindications: Not all drugs are appropriate for all people. This holds true for medicinal plants. Where research has uncovered possible negative interactions between certain physical conditions or sensitivities in a person and an herbal remedy, they are noted in this section.

Special precautions: Though many times medicinal plants may be used to treat illness without problems, there are instances where they have harmed those taking them, sometimes fatally. Overuse of plant substances has also been known to cause problems. This heading for each plant deals with special concerns noted from the research about toxicity, safety, and possible adverse reactions, particularly interactions with other drugs.

As noted earlier, plants contain numerous chemicals. Each substance, either alone or in conjunction with others, may cause allergic reactions or more severe symptoms of toxicity such as nausea, diarrhea, headaches, skin eruptions, and itching. Some dramatic examples include the cases of two patients, one in California and one in Texas, who developed cases of acute toxic hepatitis from ingesting herbal supplements from the leaves of the creosote bush, known as chaparral, according to the Centers for Disease Control. (Chaparral is a plant often mentioned as being used medicinally in the Mexican community.) In New Jersey in 1985, firefighters responding to an ambulance call of two people with severe itching themselves became stricken with the same symptoms and had to be treated after coming in contact with "voodoo beans" from the plant *Mucuna pruriens*, which grows in the Caribbean.

Mishandling and overuse of the substances may have

been a factor in each of those episodes, but the cases still serve to underscore how carefully medicinal plants have to be treated. Botanists and doctors also know that the ingestion of some plants or plant substances such as eucalyptus oil, comfrey, rue, and the essential oil of wormwood can kill. Where research has found reasons for avoiding a medicinal plant or to be cautious in its use, that information has been included.

Special mention is also made of the fact that both the experience of indigenous people in Latin America and numerous studies have shown that some plants can be abortifacients or cause menstruation. As a result, medicinal plants with those characteristics are listed so that pregnant women know which are to be avoided. A number of herbalists also have stated that pregnant and breastfeeding women, as well as children under the age of two, should not take medicinal quantities of any herbs or healing plants.

Medical research: While there may not be a great many human clinical trials of medicinal plants, scientists nevertheless have been active in probing the efficacy of plants as medicine in a variety of other experiments. The sections on medical research are aimed at encapsulating some of the findings of various studies that have focused on the usefulness of the plants as medicine and also on their toxicity. In cases where research has focused only on the chemical properties of the plants or is not available in research libraries or over the Internet, the entry will contain the notation "None noted."

There is one final important point to make. Readers using this book to further study Hispanic medicinal plants should be aware that medical research is a dynamic field, with constant changes and new findings. The research for this book was completed in late 1999, and it is always possible that in succeeding years new findings will emerge that may bring a different perspective on the efficacy and safety of the Hispanic traditional medicines listed here. For that reason, it is wise for anyone seriously considering using these plant substances to consult a physician or other medical expert for the most up-to-date information.

Traditional Hispanic Remedies and Their Historical Medical Uses

ANTI-INFLAMMATORY
Gumbo-limbo
Iporuru
Manaca
Pau d'arco
Picao preto

ARTHRITIS
Cat's claw
Chuchuhuasha
Dragon's blood
Pau d'arco

ASTHMA
Aloe vera
Amor seco
Camphor
Casca-de-anta
Chamomile

Embauba
Erva tostão
Periwinkle
Witch hazel

ASTRINGENT
Embauba
Iporuru
Quinine bark
Rhatany
Sage
Witch hazel

BRONCHITIS
Contribo
Eucalyptus

CATARRH
Anise

Balsam of Tolu
Contribo
Eucalyptus

COMMON COLD
Camphor
Contribo
Eucalyptus
Gumbo-limbo
Kalallo bush
Mozote
Oregano

COLIC (SEE GASTRO-INTESTINAL PROBLEMS)

CONSTIPATION
Copaiba
Guajava

DIARRHEA
Amargo
Amor seco
Cajueiro
Chuchuhuasha
Dragon's blood
Graviola
Guava
Iporuru
Jacote
Mozote
Mugwort

Pedra hume caa
Wormwood

DIURETIC
Annatto
Boldo
Canafistula
Chá de bugre
Erva tostão
Hierba del cancer
Picao preto
Sarsaparilla

EXPECTORANT
Avenca
Erva tostão
Thyme

GASTROINTESTINAL PROBLEMS
Anise
Basil
Boldo
Casca-de-anta
Contribo
Eucalyptus
Ginger
Graviola
Guava
Hortela (peppermint)
Jacote
Jatoba

Macela
Mugwort
Papaya
Picao preto
Rosemary

GLAUCOMA
Jaborandi

HERPES
Dragon's blood

IMPOTENCE
Muira puama

**INDIGESTION (SEE
GASTROINTESTINAL
PROBLEMS)**

INSOMNIA
Chamomile
Maracuja

LIVER PROBLEMS
Alcachofra (artichoke)
Wormwood

**MENSTRUAL PROBLEMS
(INCLUDES LATE
PERIODS OR IRREGULAR
FLOW)**
Avenca

Basil
Chuchuhuasha
Macela
Mugwort
Rue
Sage

MUSCLE ACHES
Camphor
Sour cane

ORAL HEALTH
Rhatany
Rue
Sage

PROSTATE HEALTH
Nettle

RHEUMATISM
Boldo
Cat's claw
Chuchuhuasha
Jatoba
Manaca
Pau d'arco
Sarsaparilla
Sour cane

SKIN CARE
Aloe vera
Arrowroot

Espinheira santa

Guajava

Gumbo-limbo

Pau d'arco

Espinheira santa

Guava

Macela

Quinine bark

Rosemary

STOMACHACHE (SIMPLE)

Amargo

Annatto

Basil

Boldo

Carqueja

Casca-de-anta

WOUNDS (SIMPLE)

Aloe vera

Dragon's blood

Hortela (peppermint)

Thyme

Witch hazel

❧ Alcachofra (Artichoke)

SCIENTIFIC NAME: *Cynara scolymus*

OTHER COMMON NAMES: Alcachofera, Artichaut

GROWING AREAS: Temperate areas, including parts of Mexico, Guatemala, Venezuela, and Brazil

PHYSICAL DESCRIPTION: It is a perennial herb that can grow to a height of about 6 feet. It has narrow, oblong-shaped leaves and a thick rhizome (underground horizontal stem). Its flower is used widely as a vegetable, with the petals and the bottom of the flower eaten.

TRADITIONAL USES: The artichoke is widely used in Central and South America as a medicinal plant to treat liver ailments and related problems. In Guatemala the dried leaves are reported to be sold in markets to treat liver problems, while in Brazil a decoction is used for indigestion and liver ailments. Mexicans are reported to use it for hypertension, cystitis, and calcification of the liver.

The bitterness of the artichoke is linked to phytochemicals found in the green parts of the plant. Dried artichoke leaves are useful as bitters for liqueurs.

AVAILABILITY AND DOSAGE: Powdered artichoke leaf can be purchased in capsule form. Commission E recommends a dosage of 6 grams a day.

CONTRAINDICATIONS: The product should be avoided by persons who are allergic to artichoke, as well as those with a bile duct obstruction, according to Commission E. Use by persons with gallstones is recommended only after consultation with a physician.

SPECIAL PRECAUTIONS: Consult your physician before beginning any use of an ethnobotanical substance for medicinal purposes.

MEDICAL RESEARCH: The medicinal properties of the artichoke have been attributed by research to derivatives such as cynarin and luteolin. Clinical studies have indicated that extracts from the artichoke might inhibit the body's synthesis of cholesterol and thus help persons suffering from high cholesterol levels. These studies used hepatocytes (liver cells) of laboratory rats. But a study in which cynarin doses of up to 750 milligrams a day were given to patients with high cholesterol showed no significant changes in their serum cholesterol and triglyceride levels.

Other tests performed with blood cells from rats demonstrated that extracts from the artichoke had a strong antioxidant potential and ability to protect cells from damage.

Commission E recommends the use of artichoke extract as a choleretic and to treat dyspepsia.

☙ Aloe Vera

SCIENTIFIC NAME: *Aloe barbadensis*

COMMON NAMES: Aloe Vera, Barbados Aloe, Zanzibar Aloe

GROWING AREAS: This perennial is widely available as a houseplant in the United States and grows in the tropics, including Central and South America, Mexico, India, and the Middle East.

PHYSICAL DESCRIPTION: Its leaves are green and grow in a triangular shape and taper to a point, growing to a length of 16 inches or more. The skin is tough and covered at the edges with short spines that give the leaves the appearance of serrated knife blades. Flowers produced by the plant are yellow.

TRADITIONAL USES: Among all of the botanicals used as medicine among Hispanics, the aloe vera is probably one of the best known, having found its way as a component in many health and beauty products, such as shampoo, available in the United States. But its use as a medicinal plant goes far back in history, dating to ancient Egyptian, Greek, and Mesopotamian cultures. It has become part of the Indian traditional medicine system of Ayurvedic healing. By the nineteenth century, it had also become a part of American pharmacopoeia, and by the twentieth century was being planted commercially for medicinal use.

A major use of aloe vera is as a remedy for minor burns and skin irritations because of its anti-inflammatory and wound-healing ability. It has become a staple of many kitchens, where a small piece of leaf cut from a plant and rubbed on a burn or cut can provide soothing relief. Aloe gel is obtained from the center of the blades of the plant.

In addition to its external uses, the juice of aloe vera, derived from the gel, is used as a home remedy for the treatment of asthma. Aloe vera is also used in Hispanic and other folk medicinal practices as a powerful laxative. A latex found in the plant's inner leaf skin has been used for that purpose. A substance known as aloin contained in the plant will act as a stimulant of peristaltic action in the digestive tract, causing the contractions that move food and solid waste through the alimentary tract. But in high doses, aloin will act as a powerful purgative, the effects of which can last up to twelve hours.

AVAILABILITY AND DOSAGE: Aloe is widely available as a household plant. Capsules of dried aloe vera extract or powder are also available commercially, as are aloe vera juice and gel. It is also a constituent of shampoos, skin cream, and soaps, as well as some tissues.

For topical application it can be applied liberally to wounds and burns. Though aloe vera is available in capsule form for internal use as a laxative for up to ten days, many medical experts recommend against such practice without the active involvement of a physician.

CONTRAINDICATIONS: It should not be used internally by pregnant or nursing women, or by persons with heart or kidney problems. It is also contraindicated for persons suffering from intestinal obstructions, colitis, and inflammations of the intestines.

SPECIAL PRECAUTIONS: Consult your physician before beginning any use of an ethnobotanical substance for medicinal purposes.

There is the risk of allergic reaction to aloe vera in some persons. Researchers also report that its use can delay the healing of deep wounds, including those after surgery. The powerful purgative effect of aloe vera if taken internally has prompted many doctors to warn people about never using it as a laxative or taking it internally for any purpose.

MEDICAL RESEARCH: A review of research done with laboratory animals into the antifertility aspects of certain medicinal plants showed that aloe vera was noteworthy. In one test, aloe vera leaf extract was found to inhibit the ability of rabbits to ovulate. Another test found that in laboratory rats aloe vera extract acted as an abortifacient by interfering with the ability of eggs to successfully implant within the uterus.

Numerous tests have shown the ability of aloe vera to help wounds heal, to decrease inflammation, and to relieve pain. In one study in Mexico, laboratory rats were injected in one of their feet with carrageenan, a substance that causes swelling of the paw, a condition known as "paw edema." The researchers also injected water and chloroform extracts of aloe vera gel into the paws to test for an anti-inflammatory effect. The study showed that the extracts decreased the paw edema, almost as much as commercially available anti-inflammatory substances. As a result, the researchers concluded that aloe vera gel had a potential for anti-inflammatory activity and a scientific basis for use of the plant for that purpose.

🌿 Amargo

SCIENTIFIC NAME: *Quassia amara*

OTHER COMMON NAMES: Quassia, Jamaica bark, bitter-wood, hombre grande

GROWING AREAS: Southern Mexico to Brazil

PHYSICAL DESCRIPTION: It is a shrub or small tree that can grow to a height of close to 20 feet.

TRADITIONAL USES: The bark has been widely used as a febrifuge (fever reducer) and insecticide. The plant is so bitter—more so than quinine—that extracts of it are used commercially in the production of bitters and other flavorings. Central Americans are reported to use the wood to construct clothing storage boxes that are impervious to moths.

Among the most unusual uses attributed to amargo is to treat alcoholism by mixing an extract with sulfuric acid and other substances to produce a tonic that is said to destroy the appetite for alcohol. But for the most part, it has been used as a treatment for diarrhea, particularly in Costa Rica, where indigenous peoples are said to carry around wood shavings of amargo bark to be used as needed. Brazilians also used a decoction from the wood for treating diarrhea, dysentery, and intestinal gas. Mexicans used the bark to treat intestinal parasites and a decoction made from the roots to treat stomach upset.

AVAILABILITY AND DOSAGE: It can be found in powder and capsule form. Dosages vary.

CONTRAINDICATIONS: It should be avoided by menstruating women because it may cause uterine colic, according to botanist Julia F. Morton, who lists the plant in her book *The Atlas of Medicinal Plants of Middle America*. Some experts say it is contraindicated in pregnancy.

SPECIAL PRECAUTIONS: Consult your physician before beginning any use of an ethnobotanical substance for medicinal purposes.

MEDICAL RESEARCH: Laboratory tests with male rats indicated that the plant extracts have an antifertility effect. The tests showed that an extract from the stem wood of amargo appeared to shrink the animals' testes and related organs and significantly reduced both sperm count and testosterone levels in the blood. The researchers found that the substance quassin appeared to be responsible for these effects.

🌿 Amor Seco

SCIENTIFIC NAME: *Desmodium canum*

OTHER COMMON NAMES: Strong bark, Pega Pega, Iron Vine, Amor De Campo

GROWING AREAS: Found in many tropical countries and areas ranging from southern Florida to the Caribbean, Mexico, and Paraguay, as well as Africa

PHYSICAL DESCRIPTION: It is a small shrublike plant growing about a foot tall with light purple flowers and small green fruits. Its seed pods are a little over an inch long and slightly curved, with hairs that can cling to clothing. In some countries it is found in swampy coastal areas.

TRADITIONAL USES: Traditionally it has been a popular medicinal plant in Central and South America. Indigenous tribes in Brazil have used it to treat malaria, while Nicaraguans have used it for diarrhea, venereal disease, and to aid digestion. In other parts of South America it has been used to treat nervousness, vaginal infections, and asthma, according to author Leslie Taylor.

AVAILABILITY AND DOSAGE: Available as an herbal powder for the making of decoctions as well as in tablet form. Dosages vary.

CONTRAINDICATIONS: None reported.

SPECIAL PRECAUTIONS: Consult your physician before beginning any use of an ethnobotanical substance for medicinal purposes.

MEDICAL RESEARCH: While no major clinical trials have been carried out with amor seco, a number of studies have been performed that have focused on its use as an anti-asthmatic. In one study, small doses of amor seco appeared to be helpful to asthma patients. Studies with animals showed that extracts of the plant administered orally reduced anaphylactic contractions in the bronchial area of the test subjects.

✿ Anise

SCIENTIFIC NAME: *Pimpinella anisum*

OTHER COMMON NAMES: Anise

GROWING AREAS: While rooted historically in the Mediterranean area, it is widely available in South America. Spanish colonists brought it to the New World in the sixteenth century.

PHYSICAL DESCRIPTION: An annual plant that grows to a height of up to two feet, anise puts down a long taproot and produces small white and yellow flowers, as well as a fruit that when dried out is referred to as aniseed. The aniseed is processed to produce anise oil, a volatile oil, the main constituent of which is anethole. Another variety of the plant is known as star anise (*Illicium vernum*) and is reported to have common use in Hispanic folk medicine.

TRADITIONAL USES: Anise is deeply rooted in history, and as an Old World herb was known to the ancient Egyptians and throughout the Mediterranean area. It was even mentioned in the works of Hammurabi, and botanical historians say Hippocrates recommended its use to clear the respiratory system. Dioscorides also listed it as a medicinal plant in his *De materia medica*. Its fragrance is also said to have made it valuable as a perfume. While used as a food additive—it has the taste of licorice—anise has been used medicinally as a treatment for abdominal upset and intestinal gas, as well as as a breath freshener. In medieval times, anise was used as a gargle solution with honey and vinegar to treat tonsillitis.

Within Hispanic cultures, particularly in Mexico, anise is one of the most common botanical substances used to treat colic in children.

Commission E recommends its use for dyspeptic complaints as well as for catarrhs of the respiratory system. The commission reports that it has mild antispasmodic and antibacterial properties.

AVAILABILITY AND DOSAGE: It is found in a variety of sources, including lozenges, cough drops, and teas. Anise oil is also available commercially. Commission E reports an average daily dose of 3 grams of the drug for internal use, as well as a preparation for external use of 5 to 10 percent of anise essential oil.

CONTRAINDICATIONS: Commission E reports contraindications for allergy to anise and anethole, which is found in the essential oil.

SPECIAL PRECAUTIONS: Consult your physician before beginning any use of an ethnobotanical substance for medicinal purposes.

Ingestion of anise oil has been known to cause vomiting, nausea, and pulmonary edema. Experts also caution about possible allergic reaction and contact dermatitis. Doctors and pharmacists have also warned pregnant women to steer clear of anise.

MEDICAL RESEARCH: While Commission E generally considers anise to be safe, some experts in the United States do not believe there has been adequate scientific research done to justify some of the claimed benefits attributed to it over the years. One animal study showed that anise oil had an effect on the smooth muscles of the tracheas of guinea pigs. But medical literature in the United States has not backed up the therapeutic uses of anise.

❧ Annatto

SCIENTIFIC NAME: *Bixa orellana*

OTHER COMMON NAMES: Achiote, Onoto, Achiotl

GROWING AREAS: Central and South America, as well as Mexico and the Caribbean

PHYSICAL DESCRIPTION: It is a shrub or small tree that can grow up to 30 feet tall. It is known for producing fruits covered with soft, red bristles that open when ripe to release seeds. The seeds are coated with a vermilion-colored oil. When crushed, the seeds make a red paste that is used as a food coloring and cloth dye. It also provides pigment for paints. In Belize, annatto is used to color rice red. Amazon tribes are also reported to use it for body paint and as protection from insects.

TRADITIONAL USES: Tribes in the Amazon area have used annatto as an aphrodisiac and astringent. In Brazil and Mexico it has been used as a diuretic, astringent, and purgative. It has also been used by some indigenous peoples of South America for diarrhea and dysentery. In Caribbean areas it has been used for diabetes, as a tea for removing intestinal worms, and for making a bath. Ethnobotanists also report that ingestion of the seeds of annatto has served as an antidote for certain plant poisons in Venezuela, the Amazon, and Yucatán. The pulp surrounding the seeds is used as a dye and flavoring substance.

AVAILABILITY AND DOSAGE: The powdered leaf of annatto is available in tablet or capsule form. The seeds are also sold by the pound and ounce. Some herbalists recommend taking a half cup of a decoction up to three times a day.

CONTRAINDICATIONS: None found.

SPECIAL PRECAUTIONS: Consult your physician before beginning any use of an ethnobotanical substance for medicinal purposes.

Some people have reported allergic reaction to the annatto seed, as well as a strong diuretic effect.

MEDICAL RESEARCH: There do not appear to be any clinical trials or other research on humans involving annatto. Low blood sugar has been found in dogs that have been fed extracts from the plant seeds, which may explain why some Caribbean cultures have used annatto to treat diabetic conditions. Dr. Michael Balick, a botanist with the New York Botanical Garden, has reported that in vitro testing has shown how dried ethyl alcohol extracts of the dried fruit of annatto, as well as the leaf, had an effect against two forms of bacteria troublesome to humans: *Escherichia coli* and *Staphylococcus aureus*. Both kinds of bacteria can cause gastrointestinal distress in humans. Balick also reported that an extract from the root of annatto was shown to have a smooth muscle relaxant effect on guinea pigs.

❧ Arrowroot

SCIENTIFIC NAME: *Maranta arundinacea*

OTHER COMMON NAMES: Sagu, Bermuda arrowroot, ararot

GROWING AREAS: Trinidad, Dominican Republic

PHYSICAL DESCRIPTION: Defined as an herb with a carrot-shaped, tuberous rhizome that grows to a length of 8 inches. The rhizomes are covered with a white, resinous skin coated with dry scales.

TRADITIONAL USES: As with a number of the medicinal plants used among Hispanic cultures, arrowroot is also an important food product. Starch from the plant is used widely as a foodstuff, and the rhizomes can be eaten either boiled or roasted. Arrowroot is also used in the manufacture of face powders and glue.

In terms of medicinal uses, arrowroot is believed to have received its name from indigenous peoples in Latin America who applied it to wounds from poison arrows.

In Yucatán, a poultice made from pounded arrowroot rhizomes has been used on ulcers and wounds. The rhizomes are also eaten in Yucatán for urogenital tract ailments. In Trinidad, arrowroot is used to treat sunburn and as a demulcent.

AVAILABILITY AND DOSAGE: Arrowroot is available in powder and capsule form. Dosages vary.

CONTRAINDICATIONS: None noted.

SPECIAL PRECAUTIONS: Consult your physician before beginning any use of an ethnobotanical substance for medicinal purposes.

The starch of arrowroot can produce respiratory allergic reactions.

MEDICAL RESEARCH: A pilot study by researchers in the United Kingdom found that arrowroot powder administered to eleven patients suffering from irritable bowel syndrome with diarrhea had the effect of reducing the diarrhea and easing abdominal pain.

❧ Avenca

SCIENTIFIC NAME: *Adiantum capillus-veneris*

OTHER COMMON NAMES: Maidenhair fern, maidenhair, adianto, culantrillo

GROWING AREAS: Southern United States to the Caribbean, tropical areas of Central and South America

PHYSICAL DESCRIPTION: It is a perennial herb with brown, hairy rhizomes, slender roots, and erect stems that can grow to a height of about 10 inches. Its roots are slender.

TRADITIONAL USES: In a number of areas of South America, particularly Colombia and Brazil, avenca is used as an expectorant, with a decoction made from the entire plant. In Mexico and Argentina, a decoction of the fern is reported to be used to relieve sore throat and rheumatism.

It is also reported to be used in parts of Latin America as an emmenagogue, a substance that can induce menstruation. It also has been used to hasten labor in childbirth.

AVAILABILITY AND DOSAGE: Powdered avenca leaf is available in tablets or capsules. Dosages vary. Some herbalists recommend a half cup of a decoction taken twice a day.

CONTRAINDICATIONS: None noted.

SPECIAL PRECAUTIONS: Consult your physician before beginning any use of an ethnobotanical substance for medicinal purposes.

Avenca's use in traditional medicine to stimulate menstruation presents some risk that it could cause an abortion.

MEDICAL RESEARCH: In 1989 Iraqi scientists reportedly demonstrated avenca's antimicrobial properties in a series of in vitro experiments using leaf extracts. The study showed the extract had antibacterial properties against *E. coli* and *Staphylococcus aureus*, according to the report.

It has also been reported that Belgian scientists in a study with mice determined that an avenca leaf extract had antihyperglycemic properties (i.e., prevented blood sugar from rising), according to author Leslie Taylor.

🌿 Balsam of Tolu

SCIENTIFIC NAME: *Myroxylon balsamum*

OTHER COMMON NAMES: Balsam of Peru, balsam de Peru, balsamo de Peru

GROWING AREAS: Native to southern Mexico and Panama; also cultivated in Central and South America, West Africa, and Ceylon

PHYSICAL DESCRIPTION: It is a tall tree that can grow to a height of up to 100 feet. Its bark, when cut, exudes an aromatic brown resin. The tree's flowers are fragrant and white and its leaves are evergreen.

TRADITIONAL USES: The tree is one of a number of

botanicals that were discovered by European colonists in Latin America to be useful in commerce. Legend has it that the tree was so named because the balsam was originally shipped to Spain from Callao in Peru. The balsam was so prized as incense, according to one historian, that a papal edict prohibited destruction of the tree. The balsam is obtained by injury to the tree by scoring part of the bark, which drops off and exposes the underlying wood, which then exudes the balsam. The purified balsam is then solidified. Over the years, balsam and essential oils derived from it have been used to flavor foods, soft drinks, and chewing gum.

Balsam has been used in Guatemala as a treatment for itching skin, and it is considered an irritant that sensitizes skin. In addition, Guatemalans are reported to use the dried fruit as a decoction after childbirth.

In Mexico, balsam is reported to be popular for the treatment of asthma, catarrh, and rheumatism.

On the island of Chira, off Costa Rica, the resin from the tree is used to treat toothaches by applying it to the cheek, according to Julia Morton.

AVAILABILITY AND DOSAGE: Powdered resin and bark are available in tablets or capsules. Dosages can vary. Commission E recommends 0.6 grams a day.

CONTRAINDICATIONS: None noted.

SPECIAL PRECAUTIONS: Consult your physician before beginning any use of an ethnobotanical substance for medicinal purposes.

There have been some reports of systemic toxicity in infants from the absorption of balsam after being applied to the nipples of nursing mothers to treat scabies, according to Fetrow and Avila.

MEDICAL RESEARCH: Commission E considers balsam to be useful for treating catarrh.

A study done in Greece found that balsam of Peru caused a contact dermatitis reaction in 113 of 664 patients.

Basil

SCIENTIFIC NAME: *Ocimum basilicum*

OTHER COMMON NAMES: Sweet basil, alboharcar

GROWING AREAS: Native to the Indian subcontinent; thrives in temperate and tropical zones

PHYSICAL DESCRIPTION: It is an annual herb plant that grows to a height of about 2 feet and has a squarish stem that bears many aromatic branches of about 4 inches in length.

TRADITIONAL USES: What cook does not know about basil? This aromatic herb is used in many cultures in the preparation of food. But it also has a history of medicinal use dating back to the time of the ancient Romans and Greeks. In folklore, basil has been associated with love among the Italians; a woman is said to place a pot of it on her balcony to signify she is ready to receive her lover. It has been held as sacred in India, where it has been used in burial rites.

In traditional medicine, it has been used to bring on delayed menstruation in Belize and to ameliorate painful periods, according to botanist Michael Balick. Elsewhere it has been used as an anti-inflammatory, for stomachaches, to treat intestinal parasites, and to lower blood sugar. Balick reported that it has also been used in Belize to treat earaches.

Among Mexicans on both sides of the border, it is reported to be one of the most common herbs used to treat *susto*, or gastrointestinal blockage. In the *curanderismo* ritual of *barrida*, aimed at warding off evil spirits, basil is also used as a cleansing agent, according to researchers.

AVAILABILITY AND DOSAGE: Fresh basil is readily available in food and vegetable stores, as well as *botánicas*. Dried basil is available in the spice sections of supermarkets.

Herbalists recommend using up to 3 teaspoons of dried basil leaf, or 2.5 grams, in a cup of boiling water to make an infusion for drinking. The liquid extract is also available.

CONTRAINDICATIONS: Because it is used in some cultures to promote menstruation, basil should not be used in medicinal quantity by pregnant women. It should also be used cautiously by diabetics because it is believed to lower blood sugar, which if not monitored can lead to hypoglycemia. Researchers also say it should not be given to young children or mothers who are breast-feeding.

SPECIAL PRECAUTIONS: Consult your physician before beginning any use of an ethnobotanical substance for medicinal purposes.

There are contradictory qualities attributed to basil that should be taken into consideration when its medicinal use is contemplated. While basil has been used as a medicinal plant to fight infection and to take care of gastrointestinal upset, it also contains estragol, a compound that is considered carcinogenic in animals.

MEDICAL RESEARCH: In laboratory tests, the essential oil of basil has been found to show antibacterial, antiyeast, and insecticidal action, according to Balick. A human study showed that basil significantly reduced blood glucose levels, according to Fetrow and Avila.

🌿 Boldo

SCIENTIFIC NAME: *Peumus boldus*

OTHER COMMON NAMES: Boldino, bolde

GROWING AREAS: Chile and Peru, as well as parts of Europe and North America

PHYSICAL DESCRIPTION: A common evergreen, it grows to a height of 25 feet and has leathery leaves that exude a lemon scent.

TRADITIONAL USES: Boldo is used widely in Central and South America as a medicinal tea to treat a number of gastrointestinal problems. The dried leaves are used as a mild diuretic, choleretic, and blood tonic. Chileans have used it to cure earaches as well as urogenital inflammations, including those brought on by venereal disease. Throughout Latin America, a warm bath with a leaf decoction of boldo is used for rheumatism and dropsy.

AVAILABILITY AND DOSAGE: Powdered and dried leaves are available. Commission E recommends an average dose of 3 grams of the herb that are free of ascarida. Some herbalists recommend a half cup of leaf infusion up to two times a day.

CONTRAINDICATIONS: Commission E reports that contraindications for use of boldo include obstruction of bile ducts and severe liver disease. If gallstones are present, it is recommended that boldo be used only with a physician's approval.

SPECIAL PRECAUTIONS: Consult your physician before beginning any use of an ethnobotanical substance for medicinal purposes.

James Duke says the genus *Peumus* contains the toxins pachycarpine and terpineol. The essential oil of boldo should not be used, according to Commission E.

Boldo should not be taken during pregnancy, according to Andrew Chevallier in *The Encyclopedia of Medicinal Plants*.

MEDICAL RESEARCH: In laboratory studies using animals as subjects, it was found that boldino, the major alkaloid found in the leaves and bark of boldo, acts as an antiinflammatory agent. A study in Chile in 1996 showed that administration of boldine protected rats against induced injury to the colon. The researchers believed the protection was due to the antioxidant and antiinflammatory effects of the boldine.

In another study, this time in Taiwan in 1997, researchers showed that an extract of boldine induced muscle contractions in mice.

Commission E asserts that boldine is used as a choleretic, but tests with rats did not confirm what is believed to be boldine's ability to stimulate production of bile from the gallbladder.

❧ Cajueiro

SCIENTIFIC NAME: *Anacardium occidentale*

OTHER COMMON NAMES: Cashew, caju, acajuiba, pomme cajou

GROWING AREAS: Native to Brazil; also grows in tropical areas of Central and South America, as well as the West Indies

PHYSICAL DESCRIPTION: The cashew tree grows to a height of about 25 to 30 feet with low branches. It has a rough bark. The "fruit" of the tree, known as the cashew fruit or cashew apple, is a peduncle that is fleshy and juicy. Attached to the tip of this is the cashew nut, the true fruit.

TRADITIONAL USES: In Venezuela, a decoction of the cashew leaf is used to treat diarrhea and is believed to be a treatment for diabetes. Pulverized cashew tree bark, soaked in water for twenty-four hours, is also reported to be used in Colombia for diabetes.

The juice of the false cashew fruit has been used as a diuretic in Brazil, as well as a remedy for vomiting, diarrhea, and sore throat. Peruvians also have used a tea of the cashew tree leaf as a treatment for diarrhea, while a tea from the bark has been used as a vaginal douche, said Taylor. Leaf infusions have been used to treat toothache and sore throat and as a febrifuge.

The cashew nut must be cleaned and processed to remove a toxic oil that can blister the skin.

AVAILABILITY AND DOSAGE: A 4:1 extract in powder obtained from the root is available. Dosages vary. Cashew oil is also available in *botánicas* and supermarkets for external use.

CONTRAINDICATIONS: None noted.

SPECIAL PRECAUTIONS: Consult your physician before beginning any use of an ethnobotanical substance for medicinal purposes.

The oil from the shell can cause severe dermatitis, with blistering and swelling. Even smoke from roasting cashew nuts can be irritating. Researchers have also cautioned that tannins found in the cashew bark have been documented as being toxic to humans and that the internal use of the bark must be discouraged.

MEDICAL RESEARCH: Tannins obtained from the bark of cashew trees were used in an experiment with lab rats in Brazil to test their anti-inflammatory actions. Researchers found that rats suffering from chemically induced swollen paws experienced reduced inflammation, apparently as a result of the tannins in an extract of the bark, according to the researchers. However, the study cautioned that while some folk remedies call for the use of a decoction of the cashew bark to treat rheumatism, tannins can have a toxic effect in humans and animals when taken internally.

Additional studies in India determined that extracts and oil of cashew nut shell were found to be nonmutagenic and generally did not promote tumor growth, though one aspect of the study indicated a weak tumor-promoting effect.

A study in England of plants traditionally used in northern Europe to treat diabetes mellitus determined that cashew did not affect glucose level or glucose metabolism in mice.

🌿 Camphor

SCIENTIFIC NAME: *Cinnamomum camphora*

OTHER COMMON NAMES: Alcanfor

GROWING AREAS: Once native to China, now cultivated in numerous tropical and subtropical areas

PHYSICAL DESCRIPTION: The tree is an evergreen that can grow up to 100 feet in height. Its leaves start out as red but change to a darker shade of green as the tree matures. It produces oval red berries and fragrant yellow flowers.

Camphor is obtained from the tree by steam distillation.

TRADITIONAL USES: In Puerto Rican households, camphor-based rubbing ointments are commonly used on the back and chest to treat respiratory problems such as the common cold.

In Latin America, a solution of camphor in wine used as a liniment is a folk remedy for tumors. In Mexico, according to James Duke, a mix of camphor and olive oil is popular for treating bruises and neuralgia. Camphor is also used to treat muscle aches, rheumatism, bronchitis, asthma, and lung congestion. It has been used as a rubifacient. Small doses have been taken internally for diarrhea and colds.

AVAILABILITY AND DOSAGE: Camphor is sold in *botánicas* as small, semisolid, translucent blocks. It is also contained in some well-known products such as Vicks VapoRub.

Commission E recommends external use of semisolid preparations that contain 10 to 20 percent camphor.

CONTRAINDICATIONS: Camphor can cause a burning sensation on injured skin. It is also not advisable to use it on the facial areas of small children and infants.

SPECIAL PRECAUTIONS: Consult your physician before beginning any use of an ethnobotanical substance for medicinal purposes.

Medical journals have reported cases of seizures believed to have been brought on by camphor. Contact eczema is possible when used externally. While Commission E indicates that camphor can be taken internally, a 1994 report by the American Academy of Pediatrics Committee on Drugs stated that ingestion of camphor can cause life-threatening problems. Toxic effects are said to include convulsions, dizziness, coma, and death.

MEDICAL RESEARCH: Camphor was one of a number of essential oils of plants said to be a powerful convulsant, according to one medical survey that tracked incidents involving three adults and one child who suffered from seizures. New Zealand researchers also reported the case of one twenty-month-old girl who suffered a seizure after ingesting camphor and had to be put on a ventilator. The child survived.

🌿 Canafistula

SCIENTIFIC NAME: *Cassia fistula*

OTHER COMMON NAMES: Casse, cassia, purging cassia, chacara, hojasen

GROWING AREAS: Native to South Asia, particularly India and Ceylon; cultivated widely in the tropics and as an ornamental tree in southern Florida, the West Indies, and Central and South America

PHYSICAL DESCRIPTION: *Cassia fistula* grows to a height

of about 30 feet. Its flowers are light yellow and grow in hanging clumps. The seed pods are cylindrical and have a woody brown shell up to 24 inches long, according to Julia Morton. The spaces between the seeds within the pods are filled with a sweet pulp, she said.

TRADITIONAL USES: It was given the name purging cassia in Europe during the Middle Ages and was used at that time in an Italian medical school as a purgative. In Latin America, the pulpy seed partitions have been eaten as a laxative or steeped in water for the same use. A syrup made with the flowers has also been used as a laxative.

In Guatemala, the juice of canafistula is one of several remedies used to treat urinary ailments.

AVAILABILITY AND DOSAGE: Canafistula does not appear to be available in the United States.

CONTRAINDICATIONS: Because of its reputation as a laxative, it should not be used by pregnant women.

SPECIAL PRECAUTIONS: Consult your physician before beginning any use of an ethnobotanical substance for medicinal purposes.

MEDICAL RESEARCH: In a 1987 study in Guatemala, canafistula was found to have a pronounced diuretic effect in rats.

In 1998 researchers in India began to focus on the use of canafistula to protect the liver. In a study, rats given an extract of canafistula leaf suffered less liver damage from a dose of carbon tetrachloride than rats that did not receive the extract. The effect of canafistula to reduce the damage was similar to what was observed in the use of commercially prepared drugs prescribed to treat liver problems, according to the study.

❧ Carqueja

SCIENTIFIC NAME: *Baccharis genistelloides*

OTHER COMMON NAMES: Bacanta, cacalia amara, cuchi-cuchi

GROWING AREAS: Swampy areas of Peru, Brazil, and Colombia

PHYSICAL DESCRIPTION: Carqueja is a perennial herb that grows to a height of about 20 inches. It produces a yellow flower.

TRADITIONAL USES: In traditional medicine in South America it has been used by indigenous peoples to treat sterility in women and impotence in men. It has been used to treat liver and stomach disorders, fever, sore throat, leprosy, and malaria, according to author Leslie Taylor.

AVAILABILITY AND DOSAGE: It can be found in powder and capsule forms. Dosages vary.

CONTRAINDICATIONS: None noted.

SPECIAL PRECAUTIONS: Consult your physician before beginning any use of an ethnobotanical substance for medicinal purposes.

MEDICAL RESEARCH: According to Taylor, medical studies with mice are said to show that carqueja protects the liver. One study has shown it has the ability to reduce blood sugar, while another shows it reduces gastric secretions.

In a Brazilian laboratory study, an extract of a related species was found to be active against herpes simplex type 1 virus and the virus that causes vesicular stomatitis, but not, apparently, against polio virus type 1.

🌿 Casca-de-anta

SCIENTIFIC NAME: *Drimys winteri*

OTHER COMMON NAMES: Winter's cinnamon, canelo, aktarcin

GROWING AREAS: Native to Brazil; grows in forests from southern Mexico to Cape Horn, at the very tip of Argentina; also grown as an ornamental plant in England

PHYSICAL DESCRIPTION: It is a tree that grows up to 30 feet in height. It produces a lot of small white flowers with yellow centers and a small seed pod. The flowers have a fragrant scent, like jasmine, and the seeds are fleshy and aromatic. The leaves have a peppery taste and are used as a condiment.

TRADITIONAL USES: The tree is named after Captain John Winter, who used the bark in the area of the Strait of Magellan to treat the crew of his ship, *Elizabeth*, for scurvy during the voyage of Sir Francis Drake's fleet around the world in the sixteenth century. His discovery of it as a remedy led to a great demand for the botanical in Europe.

In Brazil, according to Taylor, the bark is used as a treatment for respiratory ailments, asthma, gastrointestinal disorders such as dyspepsia, nausea, vomiting, and colic. It has sometimes been substituted for quinine to treat malaria. In Costa Rica, the bark is chewed to relieve toothaches, and an infusion is used to treat stomach disorders, said Morton.

AVAILABILITY AND DOSAGE: The bark is used as an infusion. It is not believed to be available in the United States.

CONTRAINDICATIONS: None noted.

SPECIAL PRECAUTIONS: Consult your physician before

beginning any use of an ethnobotanical substance for medicinal purposes.

MEDICAL RESEARCH: As with many botanical substances, studies done of the properties of casca-de-anta have relied on animal test subjects, not humans. But in using mice and guinea pigs, researchers in Brazil have come up with some findings that they believe point the way to further study of the plant as a human medicine, particularly in the treatment of diseases affecting the throat and lungs. In one case, mice who were suffering from a chemically induced swelling of the paw were shown to have significantly increased survival rates when given an extract of the plant. From this, the researchers concluded that the bark of casca-de-anta contained substances that had anti-inflammatory and anti-allergic properties, thus confirming its use as a folk medicine for the management of breathing problems such as asthma. In a different study, this time using guinea pigs suffering from chemically induced inflammations of the trachea, a major constituent of the bark known as polygodial was shown to interfere with constriction in the airway of the animals.

Another animal study, using mice, indicated that polygodial extracts had an antinociceptive action on animals suffering from the effects of acetic acid given internally. The acid has the effect of causing abdominal contractions, but in the test the plant extracts appeared to diminish the muscle activity, more so than aspirin and acetaminophen, two drugs used in the study for comparison.

🌿 Cat's Claw

SCIENTIFIC NAME: *Uncaria tomentosa*

OTHER COMMON NAMES: Una de gato, hawk's claw

GROWING AREAS: Peruvian rain forests of the Amazon basin, as well as Colombia, Ecuador, Guyana, Trinidad, Costa Rica, Guatemala, Panama, and Venezuela

PHYSICAL DESCRIPTION: The plant grows as a woody vine and can reach heights of around 100 feet. It earned the common name cat's claw from the claw-shaped thorns that grow from the base of the leaves. Both the bark and the root of the vine are used in the preparation of medicine. The inner bark is preferred as a medicinal source because it regenerates and its harvesting does not harm the vine.

TRADITIONAL USES: Cat's claw has a history of use going back to the time of the Incas, and it has been continuously used by indigenous peoples of South America for two thousand years. Cat's claw has been used by the Ashaninka Indians of central Peru to treat asthma, urinary tract inflammation, arthritis, and rheumatism. It has also been used by indigenous peoples to treat general inflammations and to treat wounds. In addition, some Indian peoples in Colombia are reported to use it to treat gonorrhea and dysentery.

AVAILABILITY AND DOSAGE: It can be found in liquid extract and as bark powder in capsule form. Dosages vary, though capsules can range from 25 milligrams to 500 milligrams. The raw herb can be found in cut-and-dried form in *botánicas*.

CONTRAINDICATIONS: Experts say it is contraindicated for persons undergoing skin grafts and organ transplants, as well as those suffering from coagulation disorders, tuberculosis, and autoimmune diseases.

SPECIAL PRECAUTIONS: Consult your physician before beginning any use of an ethnobotanical substance for medicinal purposes.

Experts caution that persons taking the herb should watch for signs of bleeding and possible hypotension (low blood pressure).

MEDICAL RESEARCH: Though it has been used medicinally for thousands of years, medical research into cat's claw is relatively new. Interest increased among researchers after 1970, and in 1994 the World Health Organization sponsored a conference in which cat's claw was recognized as a medicinal plant.

Researchers have focused attention on several phytochemicals in cat's claw. Among them are okindole alkaloids, found in the bark and roots, which help stimulate the immune system. Researchers have found that other alkaloids present in the plant have diuretic and hypertensive effects and lower the heart rate. Other substances found in cat's claw are believed by researchers to show antiviral and anti-inflammatory properties. Flavonoids, which are plant substances that give color to flowers and leaves, also protect the human body's cells from damage by oxidation.

The properties of cat's claw are making it useful in the study of possible treatments for AIDS, leukemia, and other forms of cancer. In mid-1999 researchers led by Alan Snow, Ph.D., of the University of Washington in Seattle announced that the National Institutes of Health were funding a study of a substance derived from cat's claw that has been found to inhibit the formation in rats of brain plaque like that associated with Alzheimer's disease. Similar effects were also found when the cat's claw substance, identified as the proprietary product PTI-00703®, was combined with another well-known botanical substance, ginkgo biloba. The results of the clinical trials are expected to be known by early 2001.

Chá de Bugre

SCIENTIFIC NAME: *Cordia salicifolia*
OTHER COMMON NAMES: Café do mato, café de bugre
GROWING AREAS: Brazil, Argentina, and Paraguay
PHYSICAL DESCRIPTION: It is a small tree that grows to a height of about 18 feet.
TRADITIONAL USES: In Brazil, according to Leslie Taylor, it is known as café do mato, "coffee of the woods," because of the red fruit produced by the plant, which resembles a coffee bean. The fruit is roasted and brewed into a tea with a high caffeine content, said Taylor. It is widely sold in pharmacies and stores in Brazil as a tea, tincture, and floral extract. It is used as an appetite stimulant, energy booster, and diuretic, most likely because of the caffeine content.
AVAILABILITY AND DOSAGE: Available as a powdered herb made from the leaf. Dosages vary.
CONTRAINDICATIONS: None noted.
SPECIAL PRECAUTIONS: Consult your physician before beginning any use of an ethnobotanical substance for medicinal purposes.
MEDICAL RESEARCH: Researchers in Japan have shown that an extract from chá de bugre inhibited the growth of

herpes simplex virus type 1, which is responsible for cold sores in humans.

🌿 Chamomile

SCIENTIFIC NAME: *Matricaria chamomilla*

OTHER COMMON NAMES: Manzanilla, English chamomile, German chamomile

GROWING AREAS: Native to Europe; grows in the United States and Central and South America

PHYSICAL DESCRIPTION: It is an annual flowering herb. *M. chamomilla* is the more widely known variety and is grown in the United States. It can reach a height of 3 feet. Another variety, Roman chamomile *(Anthemis nobilis)*, tends to grow about 8 inches high. Both varieties have flowers with small white petals and yellow centers.

TRADITIONAL USES: Of all the medicinal plants used to cure indigestion, probably none is as well known as chamomile. It has a long history of medicinal use stretching back to the time of the ancient Egyptians and Romans. Botanical historians say that the Germans have used it for centuries to treat not only stomach upset but also menstrual problems such as cramps. Doctors in England and the colony of Virginia also included chamomile in their bags of medicinals. In modern-day Eastern Europe, particularly in Romania, children were sometimes asked to bring chamomile plants to school during government-run collection campaigns.

Chamomile is believed to have been brought to the United States by immigrants from Europe, but its use has spread throughout the Hispanic cultures, where it is considered one of the key *remedios*. Considered by some to be "herbal aspirin," chamomile use is so widespread among Hispanics that one survey found it to be among the top ten substances used by mothers in Puerto Rican communities for treating asthma. In another survey done in ethnic Mexican communities along a portion of the Texas-Mexico border, chamomile was the most frequently mentioned home remedy.

Known popularly among Hispanics as manzanilla, chamomile tea is used to treat abdominal pain, vomiting, and other forms of gastrointestinal distress among children. Mexicans tend to use chamomile to treat conditions among children known as *empacho*, or blocked intestine, and *cólico*, or colic. It is also reported to be used to treat menstrual and other gynecological problems.

The traditional uses and benefits of chamomile, in both European and Hispanic cultures, have earned it a reputation for being an antispasmodic, antibacterial, deodorant, and sedative.

AVAILABILITY AND DOSAGE: It is widely available in tea form throughout the United States at the retail level. Loose chamomile flowers and crushed plants can be purchased as well for the making of teas or for use in baths. Chamomile oil is also available. Dosages vary. It is also available in capsule form in doses up to 350 milligrams.

CONTRAINDICATIONS: While Commission E said there were no known contraindications for chamomile, other researchers in the United States recommend that it should be avoided by pregnant and breast-feeding women. Caution is urged for people who are sensitive to certain volatile oils or may develop contact dermatitis.

SPECIAL PRECAUTIONS: Consult your physician before beginning any use of an ethnobotanical substance for medicinal purposes.

In their professional handbook on complementary and alternative medicines, pharmacists Charles W. Fetrow and Juan R. Avila report that chamomile is believed to be an abortifacient and should be avoided by pregnant women.

MEDICAL RESEARCH: A test done of patients undergoing cardiac catheterization showed that chamomile had no effect on heart function but put 80 percent of the patients to sleep shortly after drinking tea made from the herb.

A study done on rats determined that one of the most active substances in chamomile was bisabolol, a compound that suppresses the formation of chemically induced ulcers. Another study carried out with mice evaluated the anti-inflammatory activity of a chamomile extract. The animals' ears were chemically treated to induce swelling and then given a topical application of the extract. The chamomile extract was found to have reduced the swelling to a degree similar to that obtained with anti-inflammatory steroids.

❧ Chuchuhuasha

SCIENTIFIC NAME: *Maytenus laevis*
OTHER COMMON NAMES: Chucchu, chuchuhaso

GROWING AREAS: Areas of the Amazon basin, including Peru, Ecuador, and Colombia

PHYSICAL DESCRIPTION: It is a large tree that can grow to the height of 100 feet, creating a canopy in the forest. Its leaves can grow up to 12 inches long. It produces a small white flower.

TRADITIONAL USES: It is reported to be used by several tribes in the sub-Andean rain forest. An alcohol infusion made from the powdered root bark has been used as a tonic for treating arthritis and rheumatism and even as an aphrodisiac. Extracts from a related species *(Maytenus ilicifolia)* are reported to have been used by one tribe of indigenous people in the Amazon for birth control. Chuchuhuasha has also been used as an antitumor agent for skin cancer.

AVAILABILITY AND DOSAGE: The bark is available in powdered form. Dosages vary. Some herbalists recommend taking one cup of a bark decoction up to three times a day.

CONTRAINDICATIONS: None noted.

SPECIAL PRECAUTIONS: Consult your physician before beginning any use of an ethnobotanical substance for medicinal purposes.

MEDICAL RESEARCH: Chemicals extracted from the bark have been found by Italian researchers to have anti-tumor and anti-inflammatory effects. However, a study done by researchers in Spain showed that extracts of a related species, *Maytenus macrocarpa,* did not have any antitumor activity against human lung, colon, and melanoma cancer cells in a laboratory setting.

❧ Contribo

SCIENTIFIC NAME: *Aristolochia grandiflora*

OTHER COMMON NAMES: Duck flower, alcatraz, hierba del indio

GROWING AREAS: The southern part of Mexico to Panama

PHYSICAL DESCRIPTION: A hairy vine that grows along streams and in other wet areas. The leaves are long-stemmed and appear heart-shaped. In her encyclopedic atlas of plant life, Julia Morton has described the flower of the vine before opening as resembling the shape of a duck, with the stalk appearing like a bill and a slender tail dangling at the other end.

TRADITIONAL USES: It has a number of reported uses in Central America. Based on their studies in Central America, Michael Balick and Rosita Arvigo say that contribo is one of the most popular herbal remedies in Belize. They report that contribo can often be seen soaking in a bottle of rum at saloons, since it is taken by the shot for everything from hangovers and flu to flatulence, late menstrual periods, and irregular heartbeat. The crushed leaves are sometimes applied as a plaster for skin diseases, as a poultice for snakebite, and as an emmenagogue and treatment for diarrhea, according to Morton.

AVAILABILITY AND DOSAGE: Generally not available in the United States. In Belize, the vine is used to make a decoction or infusion.

CONTRAINDICATIONS: None noted.

SPECIAL PRECAUTIONS: Consult your physician before beginning any use of an ethnobotanical substance for medicinal purposes.

It has reportedly been used to poison humans, according to Morton. Balick and Arvigo also note that contribo contains aristolochic acid, a mutagen and carcinogen in animals, and that the use of the plant on a continuing basis "cannot be recommended." That being the case, it should be avoided.

MEDICAL RESEARCH: Balick and Arvigo reported that contribo extracts have been tested and were not found to have any antimalarial or insecticidal activity.

✣ Copaiba

SCIENTIFIC NAME: *Copaifera officinalis*

OTHER COMMON NAMES: Jesuit's balsam, copal, balsam

GROWING AREAS: Brazil, Peru, Panama, and Venezuela

PHYSICAL DESCRIPTION: It is a large tree that can grow up to 100 feet in height.

TRADITIONAL USES: The tree produces an oleoresin, which is obtained through cuts made on the bark. The resin is bitter to the taste and yellow-brown in color. In traditional medicine, the resin has been used for the treatment of bronchitis, catarrh, and inflammation of the gastrointestinal and urogenital tracts. It has also been used as a styptic for wounds and ulcers to promote healing. Though it is a plant native to Latin America, copaiba was introduced to Europe in the sixteenth century.

Copaiba has also been used for nonmedicinal purposes, such as as an additive to perfumes and varnishes.

AVAILABILITY AND DOSAGE: Available as an oil, usually sold by the ounce. Dosages vary.

CONTRAINDICATIONS: None noted.

SPECIAL PRECAUTIONS: Consult your physician before beginning any use of an ethnobotanical substance for medicinal purposes.

Researchers report that large doses can lead to vomiting, diarrhea, and skin rashes.

MEDICAL RESEARCH: Researchers in Brazil found in a 1998 study that rats fed an extract of the resin of copaiba suffered less damage to their stomach tissue from chemicals meant to induce gastric ulcers. The researchers concluded that the resin increased mucus production in the stomach and acted as an antacid.

Dragon's Blood

SCIENTIFIC NAME: *Croton lechleri*

OTHER COMMON NAMES: Sangre de draco, sangre de drago, sangre de grado

GROWING AREAS: Peru, Ecuador, and Brazil

PHYSICAL DESCRIPTION: The tree has heart-shaped, lime-colored leaves. The tree produces a red sap, hence the name dragon's blood.

TRADITIONAL USES: Peruvian Indians would extract the red sap from the tree and use it as an astringent to help heal wounds and also as a vaginal bath before childbirth. It has been used as a traditional medicine in Latin America for inflammation, cancer, and infections. The harm that can befall the tree from the harvesting of the sap has raised concern from botanists and conservationists.

AVAILABILITY AND DOSAGE: Available in liquid resin

form, as cut-and-sifted bark, and as an extract. Dosages vary.

CONTRAINDICATIONS: None noted.

SPECIAL PRECAUTIONS: Consult your physician before beginning any use of an ethnobotanical substance for medicinal purposes.

Researchers have cautioned against internal use of extracts of dragon's blood that have a high level of taspine, an alkaloid. Taspine levels can vary, depending upon the country of origin of the plant, with sap obtained from Ecuador having very little taspine but Peruvian sap having greater amounts.

MEDICAL RESEARCH: Some studies have found that the taspine, found in the red sap of dragon's blood, appears to accelerate the healing of wounds. But later research at the University of London School of Pharmacy has cast doubt on taspine's wound-healing power, suggesting instead that substances known as polyphenols may be responsible.

The same British study also examined the ability of dragon's blood to kill certain human cancer cells and bacteria. In laboratory tests on samples of human oral cancer cells, dragon's blood sap proved toxic to those cells. In addition, other components in the sap were believed to be valuable in killing off bacteria, making dragon's blood useful as an anti-infective.

A San Francisco–based firm, Shaman Pharmaceuticals, filed a patent for a dragon's-blood-based drug called Provir, based on early tests showing that 89 percent of 75 people afflicted with acute diarrhea experienced a return to normal bowel function after taking the drug. Data indicated that Provir acted by inhibiting the secretion of chloride ions from the lining of the small intestine, which tends to lead to an accumulation of fluid in that organ. This allowed Provir to treat so-called watery diarrhea, often an affliction of AIDS patients. In 1998 it was announced that trials had shown that AIDS patients who used Provir showed a significant reduction in bowel movements associated with diarrhea. In 1999 Shaman began marketing a similar product under the label SB-Normal Stool Formula as a dietary supplement.

In 1997, tests of Virend, a topical antiviral agent that Shaman derived from dragon's blood, showed that the drug reduced genital herpes lesions in AIDS patients. It appeared that Virend binds to the herpes virus and prevents it from binding to the cells of the host person, the company said. Further tests were planned.

Embauba

SCIENTIFIC NAME: *Cecropia peltata*

OTHER COMMON NAMES: Trumpet tree, trompette, imbauha

GROWING AREAS: West Indies, Mexico, Cuba, Trinidad and Tobago, Yucatán, Costa Rica, Honduras, Colombia, and Suriname; also grown as an ornamental plant in Florida

PHYSICAL DESCRIPTION: This fast-growing tree can reach up to 65 feet in height. It produces a sap described as a watery or gummy latex. Its leaves have hairy stems. The flowers develop into a spike, which in turn develops into a fleshy fruit that is soft and sweet when ripe.

TRADITIONAL USES: Cubans use the leaf as a tea for asthma and the latex as an astringent as well as a treatment for calluses and ulcers. In Guatemala, a decoction is used as a diuretic and a remedy for whooping cough. In Argentina, it has been reportedly used for Parkinson's disease. It has a wide reputation in the Caribbean as a treatment for asthma.

AVAILABILITY AND DOSAGE: Available as powdered leaf. Dosages vary. Herbalists recommend a half cup of the leaf infusion up to two times a day.

CONTRAINDICATIONS: Patients with heart conditions should not take embauba.

SPECIAL PRECAUTIONS: Consult your physician before beginning any use of an ethnobotanical substance for medicinal purposes.

It has been used to treat diabetes in Barbados. But there is a risk that blood sugar will drop too low, possibly leading to diabetic coma.

MEDICAL RESEARCH: A study in Cuba of an embauba extract showed that it had the ability to inhibit the growth of fungus.

🌿 Erva Tostão

SCIENTIFIC NAME: *Boerhaavia hirsuta*

OTHER COMMON NAMES: Pig weed, hog weed, pega-pinto

GROWING AREAS: Wide growing area stretching from the West Indies, Argentina, and Mexico to Central America

PHYSICAL DESCRIPTION: This perennial ground weed that proliferates throughout the tropics has a starchy, thick tap root. Its flowers are pink, and the seeds are coated with gummy hairs that tend to cling to people, birds, and animals, said Morton.

TRADITIONAL USES: In Latin America, it has served a number of uses, including as a treatment for asthma, as an expectorant, and as a diuretic. It is also reported to be used in Brazil as a cholagogue and as a treatment for gallstones. Researchers also report that a decoction made from the root has been used to halt uterine bleeding. For liver problems, a plaster made from powdered leaves has been placed over the area beneath which the organ lies.

In the Ayurvedic tradition of Indian folk medicine, erva tostão has been used as a diuretic and as a treatment for edema.

AVAILABILITY AND DOSAGE: It is available as a leaf powder. Dosages vary.

CONTRAINDICATIONS: None noted.

SPECIAL PRECAUTIONS: Consult your physician before beginning any use of an ethnobotanical substance for medicinal purposes.

High doses are said to cause vomiting.

MEDICAL RESEARCH: Researchers in India have tested erva tostão's use as a diuretic and anti-inflammatory. The researchers chemically induced swelling in the paws of rats and measured the reduction after an extract of the plant was given to the animals. They found a significant reduction in swelling after the extract was administered. The study also measured urine output from the animals after the extract was given and found increases in urine output.

The Indian research also found that the plant had maximal effect when the extract was taken from the roots and leaves rather than the stems. It was also determined that the time of the harvesting of the plants had an impact on the plant's medicinal effects, with maximal effectiveness if harvested during the rainy season.

Espinheira Santa

SCIENTIFIC NAME: *Maytenus ilicifolia*

OTHER COMMON NAMES: Cancrosa

GROWING AREAS: Native to Brazil; grows throughout South America

PHYSICAL DESCRIPTION: It is a small evergreen tree, resembling holly, that grows to a height of about 15 feet. Its leaves are oval-shaped and serrated.

TRADITIONAL USES: Leaves of the tree are popular as a medicine for the treatment of ulcers, dyspepsia, and other stomach problems in Brazil, where it is also reputed to be a good antacid. The *Journal of Ethnopharmacology* reports that leaves of the tree are also often used to make a tea, known as *abafado*. It is also used as a traditional contraceptive in Paraguay.

AVAILABILITY AND DOSAGE: Available as a leaf powder or as cut-and-sifted bark. Dosages vary. Herbalists also recommend a half cup of a boiled extract two or three times a day.

CONTRAINDICATIONS: None noted.

SPECIAL PRECAUTIONS: Consult your physician before beginning any use of an ethnobotanical substance for medicinal purposes.

Though tests on animals for toxicity showed no adverse effects, the plant did act as a significant sedative and might, if used by humans in significant amounts, accentuate the effect of other drugs that can cause drowsiness, such as antihistamines.

MEDICAL RESEARCH: A number of tests have been done in Brazil on laboratory animals to test the anti-ulcer effects of the plant, as well as its possible toxicity, with what appear to be encouraging results. One test, using rats who were given a chemical to induce a gastric ulcer, showed that a water extract of dried *Maytenus* leaves increased the pH of the gastric juices of the animals, thus making the stomachs less acidic and better able to resist tissue damage. These results thus confirm the popular use of this plant. Another study in rats and mice found that different doses, including some that were four hundred times those used by humans, did not appear to have any toxic effect on the mice, nor did the plant impact the animals' fertility. High doses of the plant preparation did act as a sedative when given by injection. However, the overall results led researchers to conclude that *Maytenus* may be a safe plant for human use and deserving of further investigation.

But not so promising have been tests performed on cancer patients in the United States of the compounds, maytansine and mayteine that are found in the plant. While there was some effect seen on ovarian cancer and some lymphomas with maytansine, the substance was deemed toxic at the higher doses that were needed to be used, according to a report in a medical journal.

Eucalyptus

SCIENTIFIC NAME: *Eucalyptus globulus*

OTHER COMMON NAMES: Australian fever tree, euca-
lypto, eucalypt

GROWING AREAS: Native to Australia; also grows in the
Mediterranean area and South America

PHYSICAL DESCRIPTION: It is a fast-growing tree that
can reach 400 feet in some areas.

TRADITIONAL USES: When the eucalyptus tree was first
planted in the Mediterranean, it gained a reputation as
an antimalarial plant—primarily, it seems, because it
absorbed a great deal of water through its roots and effectively dried up swamps and waterways where mosqui-
toes bred. The oil of the leaves, which has a distinctive
aroma similar to camphor, has been used in many cultures to treat colds, flu, bronchitis, and catarrh, mainly
because of the way it can open up bronchial tubes and
relieve congestion. It is considered to be an expectorant
and weak antispasmodic, for which it has been reported
to be used in Turkey. It is widely used in South America
to treat respiratory infections and as a rubefacient, a
substance that increases blood flow to the skin. Some
herbalists say it is also an effective treatment for small
cuts on the skin. Others report that a piece of cloth
soaked in the oil can repel cockroaches.

Commission E has labeled eucalyptus as an expectorant, secretomotory, and mild antispasmodic. It is used
in small amounts in over-the-counter cold and cough
remedies.

AVAILABILITY AND DOSAGE: Available in *botánicas* in
the form of dried leaves and also as a volatile oil pre-

pared from the leaves through a distillation process. Some herbalists recommend boiling a few leaves or a few drops of essential oil in water as an inhalant. For minor cuts, a drop or two of essential oil rubbed on the affected area is sometimes recommended by herbalists.

CONTRAINDICATIONS: Women who are pregnant or breast-feeding, as well as anyone suffering from low blood sugar (hypoglycemia). Commission E says it is contraindicated for persons suffering from inflammatory diseases of the gastrointestinal tract, liver, and bile ducts, as well as severe liver disease.

SPECIAL PRECAUTIONS: Consult your physician before beginning any use of an ethnobotanical substance for medicinal purposes.

Despite the fact that it is widely used to treat respiratory infections and catarrh, eucalyptus has to be treated with care. If taken internally, eucalyptus oil can cause nausea and vomiting and can even be fatal. It may on occasion cause skin irritation. Researchers have also noted that essential oil from eucalyptus can be a powerful convulsant and may prompt seizures. Commission E recommends that it not be used on the faces of babies and young children, probably because it might be ingested. Commission E also says eucalyptus stimulates the enzyme system of the liver involved in the detoxification process and as a result can weaken or alter the effects of other drugs.

MEDICAL RESEARCH: Tests done in Guatemala of a number of plants used for the treatment of respiratory ailments examined their antibacterial activity on commercially prepared strains of bacteria, including those that cause pneumonia and staphylococcus infections. The test results

showed that extracts of *Eucalyptus globulus* were among
the plants shown to be highly active against the bacteria
during the in vitro tests. However, further tests on humans
were needed to examine the properties of the extract, according to the researchers.

✺ Ginger

SCIENTIFIC NAME: *Zingiber officinale*

OTHER COMMON NAMES: Gengibre, gingembre

GROWING AREAS: China, Jamaica, southwestern parts of
the United States, Hawaii

PHYSICAL DESCRIPTION: Ginger is a perennial plant that
produces a thin stem about 3 feet long, with leaves
that are thin and pointed. It produces a purple flower
that looks like an orchid. Its thick rhizome is the most
important part of the plant.

TRADITIONAL USES: Ginger has been recognized as an
important plant in Chinese medicine for centuries and is
mentioned in two-thousand-year-old medical books. It
was valued for its medicinal and culinary uses, serving
as both a seasickness remedy for sailors and a pungent-
tasting condiment. The ability of ginger to act as an
antiemetic, a substance that relieves stomach upset, has
been a key to its use by humans over the centuries. It is
also used to treat diarrhea, nausea, and arthritis, and as
an appetite stimulant. It is widely used in Jamaica,
Mexico, and India for medicinal and other purposes, including as a spice and in beverages and candies.

AVAILABILITY AND DOSAGE: Ginger is widely available
in the United States as a liquid extract, powder, tablets,

and capsules. Gingerroot and ginger tea can also be obtained in food stores. Dosages vary, and some herbalists maintain that a 12-ounce glass of ginger ale, assuming it is made from real ginger, will have the same remedial effect on motion sickness that a 1,200-milligram dose of powder has.

CONTRAINDICATIONS: Some experts recommend that it not be used, except under medical supervision, by people who are receiving anticoagulants. They also caution against pregnant women using ginger.

SPECIAL PRECAUTIONS: Consult your physician before beginning any use of an ethnobotanical substance for medicinal purposes.

In their professional handbook on alternative and complementary medicine, Juan R. Avila and Charles W. Fetrow, both pharmacists, say there is no consensus on what the proper dosage is for ginger. They also advise pregnant women not to use it.

MEDICAL RESEARCH: A great deal of the research into ginger and its medicinal properties has focused on its antiemetic and antinausea effects. According to a study published in the British medical journal *Lancet*, ginger seemed to be more effective than some standard drugs in treating motion sickness and dizziness. According to the *Lancet* results, volunteers who took ginger were able to endure artificially created seasickness (from a mechanical rocking chair) 57 percent longer than those who used Dramamine.

Ginger is also seen as being useful for controlling and relieving the nausea that can result from cancer chemotherapy. Researchers in India in 1997 tested the ability of ginger extract to alleviate the gastrointestinal distress associated with chemotherapy. The researchers fed laboratory rats an extract of ginger in varying doses before giving the animals cisplatin, an anticancer chemical. The test results showed that ginger was able to increase the rate at which the rats' stomachs emptied, leading the researchers to conclude that ginger may relieve the abdominal symptoms associated with chemotherapy.

Additional studies using acetone extracts of ginger in laboratory rats showed that two constituents of the plant, known collectively as gingerol, were responsible for increased bile production in the animals. This indicated that extracts of gingerroot can play an important role in digestion and food absorption.

Graviola

SCIENTIFIC NAME: *Annona muricata*

OTHER COMMON NAMES: Guanabana, guanavana, guanaba, anona de broquel

GROWING AREAS: Said to be native to the West Indies; has spread from southern Mexico to Brazil

PHYSICAL DESCRIPTION: It is a tall, slender tree that grows to a height of about 24 feet. The leaves, which stay evergreen in tropical areas, are dark green and glossy. When crushed, the leaves give off a strong odor. The fruit is described as heart-shaped with a green skin that is covered with spines. The inner flesh of the fruit is juicy and aromatic and has numerous black seeds, according to Julia Morton.

TRADITIONAL USES: Graviola is a plant that has many

medicinal uses in folk traditions but has to be used cautiously, as noted below in the discussion of special precautions. In Panama and Venezuela it is reported to be used to treat diarrhea, while Mexicans use it for fever and dysentery and as an astringent. Researchers also note that it is used to combat a number of gastrointestinal ailments in Puerto Rico, where it is used as an antispasmodic, antidiarrheal, and stomachic. Julia Morton reported that graviola is a popular bush tea in the Caribbean and Bahamas, where it is sweetened and consumed by children and adults. It is also in the Caribbean that graviola is used to treat colds and fever, according to Morton.

AVAILABILITY AND DOSAGE: Available in powdered leaf form. Dosages vary. Herbalists recommend that a half cup of the leaf infusion be taken one to three times daily.

CONTRAINDICATIONS: None noted.

SPECIAL PRECAUTIONS: Consult your physician before beginning any use of an ethnobotanical substance for medicinal purposes.

Though it is widely used in the Caribbean and in parts of Latin America, *Annona muricata* is considered by some doctors and researchers to be a potentially toxic plant. Its seeds are reported to be toxic and have been used as an insecticide and fish poison. In fact, parts of the fruit and a decoction from the leaves are reported to be used as a vermifuge in the Caribbean. Perhaps more troubling are results of tests showing that leaf extracts from the plant injected into rats produced fibrosarcomas in one-third of the animals at the point of injection, something researchers attributed to the high tannin content of the extract.

MEDICAL RESEARCH: *Annona muricata* was one of twelve
medicinal plants tested by researchers in Brazil examin-
ing the analgesic effects of popular folk remedies. The researcher administered extracts from the plants to the
animals and tested their reaction to stimulus. They
found that *Annona muricata* was virtually inactive as an
analgesic but that all of the animals receiving it died
within twenty-four hours.

✿ Guajava

SCIENTIFIC NAME: *Cassia alata*

OTHER COMMON NAMES: Date, candle tree, ringworm
cassia

GROWING AREAS: Widely available in the tropics; said to
be native to the West Indies, as well as southern Mexico
and parts of South America

PHYSICAL DESCRIPTION: It is a shrub that can grow up
to 12 feet high. It has yellow flowers that grow in clusters
and are said to resemble candles because of the way
they stand.

TRADITIONAL USES: It is used in Mexico, Venezuela, and
the Dominican Republic as a diuretic. It has also been
given the name ringworm cassia because a leaf extract is
used to combat ringworm and is sometimes put into
bathwater for that purpose, particularly in Malaysia. In
Guatemala, Suriname, and Mexico it is used to relieve
constipation. The leaves have been reported to treat ulcers and other skin diseases.

AVAILABILITY AND DOSAGE: Available as a powdered
leaf. Dosages vary.

CONTRAINDICATIONS: None noted.

SPECIAL PRECAUTIONS: Consult your physician before beginning any use of an ethnobotanical substance for medicinal purposes.

In studies done on patients suffering constipation, it has caused some diarrhea, abdominal pain, and nausea. It also has a reputation in South American traditional medicine as being able to act as an abortifacient or stimulant that could promote menstruation.

MEDICAL RESEARCH: Some studies involving human subjects have pointed to beneficial effects attributed to the plant. In a clinical study done in India, extracts from *Cassia alata* were investigated for their effectiveness as antifungal compounds. In a test on patients with confirmed cases of a fungus infection on the skin known as *Pityriasis versicolor*, a fresh extract from the leaves of *Cassia alata* was applied to infected areas one time and washed off the next morning. The study found that the infected areas began to clear up in three weeks and led to what the researchers believe was a cure for up to a year, after which a relapse occurred. The findings, along with the lack of any side effects, led to the conclusion that *Cassia alata* is an effective, reliable, and safe herbal medicine for treating this particular skin ailment.

However, a Malaysian study found that an extract of *Cassia alata* had no effect in the laboratory on a number of microorganisms, including bacteria and yeast, that cause skin diseases in humans. The extract did have some effect on fungus growth, but researchers could not say with certainty how it occurred.

A study of hospital patients in Bangkok suffering from constipation was reported to have determined that an extract of *Cassia alata* was an effective laxative, providing relief, often within twenty-four hours, with a return of bowel movements in over 86 percent of the patients. The researchers attributed the laxative effect to the substance in the plant known as anthraquinones. However, it was also noted that a number of the patients complained of side effects, including diarrhea, abdominal pain, and nausea.

Cassia alata has been reputed in folklore to act as an abortifacient or promote menstruation. But in tests done on female laboratory rats in Brazil, *Cassia alata* did not show such traits.

 Guava

SCIENTIFIC NAME: *Psidium guajava*

OTHER COMMON NAMES: Guayaba, guayava, guayabo casero

GROWING AREAS: Native throughout Latin America

PHYSICAL DESCRIPTION: It is a shade tree that grows to about 30 feet, has a red flaky bark, and produces a very aromatic fruit with a yellow skin and dark pink edible flesh. The inner pulp of the fruit is soft and contains many yellow seeds.

TRADITIONAL USES: Guava is one of a number of plants that do double duty in Hispanic communities. As a food source, it is widely consumed and used in beverages and desserts. The fruit is high in ascorbic acid. European traders spread the fruit to Asia and Africa. The tree's bark is used in the tanning of animal skins, and the wood can be used in construction.

Guava has been widely used in Latin American traditional medicine as a treatment for diarrhea and stomachaches due to indigestion. Treatment usually involves drinking a decoction of the leaf, roots, and bark of the plant. It also has been used for dysentery in Panama and as an astringent in Venezuela. A decoction of the plant's bark and leaves is also reported to be used as a bath to treat skin ailments.

AVAILABILITY AND DOSAGE: Guava is readily available in food stores, *botánicas*, and bodegas throughout Hispanic and non-Hispanic communities in the United States. Dosages vary.

CONTRAINDICATIONS: None noted.

SPECIAL PRECAUTIONS: Consult your physician before beginning any use of an ethnobotanical substance for medicinal purposes.

The seeds of the guava fruit have been labeled as digestion-resistant by researchers, which explains how the seeds are dispersed by animals and humans. Guava has also been shown to have the ability to lower blood sugar, but blood sugar levels that are too low can be dangerous, with the risk of disorientation, coma, and even death.

MEDICAL RESEARCH: There have been a number of laboratory studies done on guava, mainly as a way of controlling noninfectious diarrhea, long a significant cause of infant mortality in developing countries. Studies have shown that extracts of dried guava leaves can slow down peristalsis (movement of food through the digestive tract), which increases absorption of fluid and electrolytes and thus reduces both diarrhea and the dehydration it can cause.

In traditional medicine, guava has also been used to

lessen pain, combat insomnia, and help children suffering from convulsions, properties that sparked more scientific inquiry. Additional studies done in Malaysia, where the plant grows abundantly, showed that an extract of dried guava leaves had a narcoticlike effect on rats, something researchers attributed to flavonoids present in the plant.

Some of the flavonoids present in guava leaves are also viewed by researchers as having potential antitumor properties. A study done in Mexico used guava leaf extracts in a laboratory setting and found that it showed significant activity against certain human and mouse cancer cell lines.

Chinese and Caribbean traditional medicine have used guava in the control of diabetes, but a study in Mexico found that guava did not lower blood sugar levels in rabbits.

Gumbo-limbo

SCIENTIFIC NAME: *Bursera simaruba*

OTHER COMMON NAMES: Jobo, almacigo, desnudo

GROWING AREAS: Native to the Amazon area, Belize, elsewhere in Central America, and parts of tropical South America; also reported to be native to Florida

PHYSICAL DESCRIPTION: It is a tree that can grow to about 60 feet. The bark is distinctive, peeling off in thin strips. Botanist Michael Balick of the New York Botanical Garden, an expert on plants in Belize, said the tree has a fragrant yellow-green flower and a fruit that is round and tinged with red.

TRADITIONAL USES: Botanists report that it is used in Belize as a treatment for dermatitis and irritations from poisonwood sap, mainly by immersion of the skin in a cool tea made from the bark of the tree. Balick reported that the same bark bath has been used to treat discomfort from insect bites, sunburn, measles, and other skin problems. Venezuelans are reported to use it externally as an ointment to treat rheumatism. Used internally in traditional medicine in South America, it is believed to be helpful in fighting colds, urinary tract infections, and the flu.

In Costa Rica, the plant is used as a traditional treatment for gastric cancer, with anecdotal reports that it relieves discomfort from that illness. It is one of a number of medicinal plants in that country undergoing screening to determine if it contains substances that might be useful in fighting stomach cancer.

In her study of medicinal plants of Belize, Jane Mallory says that the resin of *Bursera simaruba* is painted on boats to protect the wood from worms and insects. The wood is also used for everything from matchsticks to the construction of crates.

AVAILABILITY AND DOSAGE: Available as a powdered leaf. Dosages vary.

CONTRAINDICATIONS: None noted.

SPECIAL PRECAUTIONS: Consult your physician before beginning any use of an ethnobotanical substance for medicinal purposes.

An extract of the bark of the tree is reported to be effective at killing snails.

MEDICAL RESEARCH: Since gumbo-limbo is considered to have anti-inflammatory qualities, researchers in Venezuela tested the effects of an extract of gumbo-limbo tree bark on laboratory rats with induced swelling of the hindpaw and an arthritic knee joint. The extract caused a significant reduction in the paw swelling as well as inflammation of the arthritic knees in the test animals. The researchers speculated that the results were attributable to a suppression of the animals' immunological response in general but cautioned that further experiments were needed.

🌿 Hierba del Cancer

SCIENTIFIC NAME: *Acalypha guatemalensis* Pax & Hoffman, *Acalypha arvensis* Poepp & Enbdl.

OTHER COMMON NAMES: Petit mouton, bonda pe, petit pompon, cat tail

GROWING AREAS: Native to Central America

PHYSICAL DESCRIPTION: An herb that grows up to 3 feet in height. The leaves are long-stemmed and oval-shaped.

TRADITIONAL USES: According to Balick and Arvigo, the common name hierba del cancer stems not from the ability of the plant to fight cancer but rather because of the local use of the word *cancer* to mean an open sore. They report that the plant is used as a remedy in Belize for a variety of serious skin conditions such as fungus, ulcers, ringworm, and itching or burning labia in women. It is one of scores of plants used throughout Latin America as a diuretic. The leaves are used in Guatemala not only as a diuretic but also to treat kidney-related problems. In Haiti it is used to treat diarrhea, inflammations, and dyspepsia.

AVAILABILITY AND DOSAGE: Not available in the United States.

CONTRAINDICATIONS: None noted.

SPECIAL PRECAUTIONS: Consult your physician before beginning any use of an ethnobotanical substance for medicinal purposes.

MEDICAL RESEARCH: In a study of plants used in Guatemala as diuretics and for the treatment of urinary ailments, extracts of hierba del cancer were shown to increase urinary output by 30 percent.

Balick and Arvigo report that studies have shown a dried leaf tincture to be active against *Staphylococcus aureus* but inactive against some other bacteria. They also noted that extracts of dried twigs were found to be inactive against human colon cancer cells in vitro.

Hortela (peppermint)

SCIENTIFIC NAME: *Mentha piperita*

OTHER COMMON NAMES: Menta, mentha montana

GROWING AREAS: Thought to have originated in the Middle East; grows in tropic and temperate zones around the world

PHYSICAL DESCRIPTION: A perennial plant, *Mentha piperita* grows to a height of about 2 feet. It has a squarish stem and leaves that are serrated on the edges. It produces a light purple flower in the summer months. It also produces rhizomes, which are used for cultivating additional plants.

TRADITIONAL USES: Peppermint is widely used in traditional medicine around the world as a digestive aid, having a long history of such use dating back to the Roman era. Historians say it was also used in the ancient world to prevent the spoilage of milk.

In modern herbal practice, *Mentha piperita* is used to treat colic, indigestion, and colds, as well as minor wounds and burns. Some experts say it is used by women to bring on menstrual flow. Among Hispanics, another member of the mint family, spearmint, is used as a home remedy to treat colic, diarrhea, and upper respiratory tract infections. Mexicans use varieties of mint to treat children for the folk illness known as *empacho* or blocked intestine.

Commission E lists both the leaf and oil of peppermint among the plant substances deemed acceptable for human consumption. The commission reports that peppermint leaf acts as an antispasmodic on the smooth muscles of the digestive tract and is useful as a cholagogue. Peppermint oil, obtained from the stem of the plant by a distillation process, is also used for treating discomfort of the upper gastrointestinal tract and bile ducts, as well as for catarrh and inflammations of the mucous membranes of the mouth, the commission stated.

AVAILABILITY AND DOSAGE: Peppermint is available as an essential oil and in leaf form in health food stores and *botánicas*. The essential oil is also available in enteric-coated pill form.

Commission E recommends a dose of 6 to 12 drops a day of peppermint oil for internal use or 0.6 milliliters in enteric-coated capsules daily for irritable colon. For inhalation, 3 or 4 drops of essential oil in hot water is recommended. However, other experts say there is no consensus for the oil's internal use and recommend against taking it in that fashion. An infusion can be made by pouring half a cup of hot water over a teaspoon of the dried pulverized herb.

Peppermint is also available as a tea, either on its own or in combination with other herbs. Menthol, the major component of peppermint oil, is used in lozenges, sprays, and other cold and cough remedies. Menthol is also available in creams and skin ointments for external use as an analgesic.

CONTRAINDICATIONS: Commission E notes that peppermint oil should not be used without a doctor's permission in individuals with obstructions of the gallbladder, gallstones, or severe liver disease. The commission states the same caution for peppermint leaf in cases of gallstones. Experts also caution against pregnant women using strong infusions of peppermint, undoubtedly because it is reputed to stimulate menstruation.

SPECIAL PRECAUTIONS: Consult your physician before beginning any use of an ethnobotanical substance for medicinal purposes.

Peppermint and menthol are reported to have caused allergic reactions in some adults and children, the latter sometimes known to suffer gagging reflexes. Doctors also warn about applying peppermint oil or products containing it to broken skin. The PDR for Herbal Medicine states that doses of menthol as low as 2 grams can be lethal, although some survive doses as high as 9 grams.

MEDICAL RESEARCH: Peppermint and menthol have been the subject of a number of studies by medical researchers. Peppermint has been found in some studies to have an antiviral effect, which may explain its usefulness as a cold remedy. As noted, peppermint is also reported to act as an antispasmodic on certain smooth muscles in the gastrointestinal tract, an effect that researchers believe stems from the way it interferes with the flow of calcium into muscle cells. Other studies have shown that menthol helps to dissolve gallstones.

🌿 Iporuru

SCIENTIFIC NAME: *Alchornea floribunda*

OTHER COMMON NAMES: Iporuro, niando, iporoni

GROWING AREAS: The floodplains of the Amazon in Peru

PHYSICAL DESCRIPTION: Iporuru is an evergreen shrub.

TRADITIONAL USES: Among indigenous Amazonian tribes, the genus is used to treat rheumatism and arthritis. Its perceived anti-inflammatory properties have made iporuru popular in North America as a treatment for arthritis and rheumatism, according to author Leslie Taylor. It is also a plant cultivated in Africa, where it is reported to be used for gonorrhea and coughs.

James Duke reported that the macerated root has been used as a strong intoxicant and aphrodisiac.

AVAILABILITY AND DOSAGE: Available as a leaf powder. Dosages vary. Herbalists recommend taking one half cup of a leaf infusion one to three times a day.

CONTRAINDICATIONS: None noted.

SPECIAL PRECAUTIONS: Consult your physician before beginning any use of an ethnobotanical substance for medicinal purposes.

MEDICAL RESEARCH: A study found that an extract of the bark of a related species appeared to act as an antispasmodic and an antibacterial agent and is thus useful in combating diarrhea.

🌿 Jaborandi

SCIENTIFIC NAME: *Pilocarpus jaborandi*

OTHER COMMON NAMES: Indian hemp, pernambuco, arruda brava

GROWING AREAS: Northern parts of Brazil

PHYSICAL DESCRIPTION: It is a shrub about 5 feet high with large, feathery leaves.

TRADITIONAL USES: *Pilocarpus jaborandi* is one of a number of medicinal plants from the Amazon that have found their way into the mainstream of the medical profession. Explorers to Brazil as far back as the sixteenth century discovered that indigenous tribes used the plant to treat mouth ulcers, colds, and flu. Samples of the plant were eventually taken to Peru, where researchers discovered that it was able to promote sweating and salivation in humans. After continued research, the alkaloid pilocarpine was identified in the plant; this substance has the ability to lower pressure within the eye of a person with glaucoma. As a result of that finding, pilocarpine is used in modern ophthalmology as a treatment for glaucoma.

Pilocarpus jaborandi is recorded as being used to treat rheumatism, pleurisy, and dropsy in Mexican traditional medicine. It is also said to have a history of use as an emetic in Brazil.

AVAILABILITY AND DOSAGE: Not generally available.

CONTRAINDICATIONS: In their professional handbook on

alternative and complementary medicine, Charles Fetrow and Juan R. Avila say that pilocarpine is contraindicated for persons sensitive to it, as well as those with uncontrolled asthma.

SPECIAL PRECAUTIONS: Consult your physician before beginning any use of an ethnobotanical substance for medicinal purposes.

Because of risk of toxic symptoms such as excessive sweating, fast heart rate, and salivation, the use of jaborandi should be undertaken only with the advice and participation of a doctor.

MEDICAL RESEARCH: None noted.

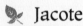 Jacote

SCIENTIFIC NAME: *Spondia mombin*

OTHER COMMON NAMES: Jobo, job megro, ciruela de jobo, Spanish plum

GROWING AREAS: Native to Southeast Asia and Malaysia; cultivated throught the West Indies, as well as much of Mexico and the rest of Latin America

PHYSICAL DESCRIPTION: This tree can reach 60 feet or higher. It has fragrant red flowers. Its fruit, which are oblong, red or yellow, and fragrant and contain a juicy and acidic pulp, hang in clusters from the tree.

TRADITIONAL USES: In traditional medicine of Latin America, jacote has many uses for a wide range of illnesses. Brazilians use the bark to make a decoction for the treatment of diarrhea, while a decoction from the flowers and leaves is reportedly used to relieve constipation and stomachache. Famed ethnobotanist Richard

Schultes reports that the Tikunas Indians of the Amazon area use a decoction of the bark to relieve pain and to prevent excessive bleeding during menstruation. He says they also use it to treat stomach pains and diarrhea as well as as a wash for wounds. According to Julia Morton, Cubans have traditionally eaten large amounts of the fruit as an emetic, while Haitians take the fruit syrup as a remedy for angina. Mexicans use it to treat diarrhea, while Dominicans have used it as a laxative. Its bark also has a reputation in folk medicine for being useful in treating minor skin ulcers.

The fruit is eaten as a food and can be made into jellies and preserves. The wood is used in the manufacture of crates and other light items.

AVAILABILITY AND DOSAGE: It can be purchased through mail-order herbal suppliers in Central America.

CONTRAINDICATIONS: None noted.

SPECIAL PRECAUTIONS: Consult your physician before beginning any use of an ethnobotanical substance for medicinal purposes.

Schultes reports the Amazon Indian belief that "permanent sterility" would result from the drinking of one cup a day of a decoction of jacote following childbirth. According to Morton, Colombians believe the fruit is bad for the throat and that the leaves and bark contain tannin and thus are astringent.

MEDICAL RESEARCH: None noted.

🌿 Jatoba

SCIENTIFIC NAME: *Hymenaea courbaril*

OTHER COMMON NAMES: Courbaril, pois confiture, stinking toe, azucar huayo, West Indian locust

GROWING AREAS: Native to Peru and Brazil; also grows in Central America

PHYSICAL DESCRIPTION: This tree can reach 60 feet or higher and has a trunk that can be over 6 feet in diameter. The base of the tree emits an odorless resin that is found in great quantities around the roots. Its fruit is reddish and oblong with a difficult-to-crack, woody surface. The pulp of the fruit is described by Julia Morton as "odorous, sweet, dry, mealy, buff-colored."

TRADITIONAL USES: In the Virgin Islands, *Hymenaea courbaril* is reported to be used as an infusion with blood-purifying properties. Julia Morton reports that it is used in Central America as a vermifuge, as a remedy for hypertension and rheumatism, and as a substitute for quinine, apparently to fight malaria. She reported that the bark decoction has been used to treat diarrhea, dysentery, stomach ulcers, and chest ailments. Fumes of the burning resin, Morton says, have been used in Mexico to relieve asthma and "hysteria."

The fruit is also eaten as a food, and the wood is hard enough to use in carpentry, said Morton.

AVAILABILITY AND DOSAGE: Available as a cut-and-sifted bark powder. Dosages vary. Herbalists recommend a half cup of the decoction three times daily.

CONTRAINDICATIONS: None noted.

SPECIAL PRECAUTIONS: Consult your physician before

beginning any use of an ethnobotanical substance for medicinal purposes.

MEDICAL RESEARCH: According to Morton, the high tannin content of the leaves has shown activity against a form of lung cancer in mice during experiments.

🌿 Kalallo Bush

SCIENTIFIC NAME: *Corchorus siliquosus*

OTHER COMMON NAMES: Hiera te, malva te, te de la tierra

GROWING AREAS: Native to the Virgin Islands and West Indies; also found in Mexico and Central America

PHYSICAL DESCRIPTION: A bush about 3 feet high with short-stemmed leaves. The flowers are yellow and the seed capsule is flat.

TRADITIONAL USES: A decoction of this plant is reported to be used frequently in Central America as a refreshing drink. In the Virgin Islands the plant is cooked and eaten and used as a treatment for colds. It has been used as a treatment for venereal disease in Yucatán and for bladder trouble and as a bathwater additive in Cuba, according to Julia Morton.

AVAILABILITY AND DOSAGE: The product is not believed to be available in the United States.

CONTRAINDICATIONS: None noted.

SPECIAL PRECAUTIONS: Consult your physician before beginning any use of an ethnobotanical substance for medicinal purposes.

MEDICAL RESEARCH: None noted.

🌿 Macela

SCIENTIFIC NAME: *Achyrocline satureoides*

OTHER COMMON NAMES: Juan blanco, macela do campo, marcela hembra

GROWING AREAS: Native to Venezuela and parts of the Brazilian Amazon as well as Central America

PHYSICAL DESCRIPTION: It is an aromatic shrub that grows to a height of about 3 feet. It has flowers that are small and yellowish or white. The seeds are oval-shaped and bristled.

TRADITIONAL USES: Macela has a well-respected reputation in South America as a medicinal plant useful in the treatment of gastrointestinal problems and inflammations. In Venezuela it is reported to be used as an emmenagogue and in Brazil as cough medicine. Argentines also have used it as an emmenagogue and to treat vaginal infections.

AVAILABILITY AND DOSAGE: Available in powdered leaf form. Dosages vary. Herbalists recommend a half cup of the leaf infusion once or twice daily.

CONTRAINDICATIONS: None noted.

SPECIAL PRECAUTIONS: Consult your physician before beginning any use of an ethnobotanical substance for medicinal purposes. It has been used as an emmenagogue.

MEDICAL RESEARCH: A number of laboratory experiments have demonstrated that macela extracts have been useful in treating artificially induced inflammations in rats. Additional studies have shown the flavonoids present in macela to have analgesic and antispasmodic properties, as well as having an effect on constipation.

In a Brazilian study aimed at evaluating macela's anti-inflammatory properties, the ears of laboratory mice were irritated with the application of croton oil. For each test animal, one swollen ear was treated with the topical application of an extract of macela, while the other was left untreated. Five hours into the experiment, and at the height of the irritation, the animals were sacrificed and small disks were punched out of both ears and weighed. Researchers assumed the difference in the weight of the ears would be an indication of the response of the swelling to the plant extract. The results indicated that a water extract showed the greatest reduction of the swelling (by 41 percent). As a result, the researchers believed the tests supported the use in folk medicine of macela in the treatment of inflammatory diseases.

Tests have also been done with macela extracts showing that in laboratory settings it has been effective in killing the parasites that cause trypanosomiasis in humans, as well as other microorganisms.

❧ Mallow

SCIENTIFIC NAME: *Malvestrum sylvestris*

OTHER COMMON NAMES: Malva, malva grande, malva real

GROWING AREAS: Native to much of South and Central America

PHYSICAL DESCRIPTION: It is a bush herb that grows to a height of 3 feet and generally is found at low elevations. Its stem has been described as stiff with hair, and its leaves have sharp teeth on the edges. Its flowers are reddish purple, and its flat fruit produces seeds that are shaped like kidney beans.

The mucilage contained in the leaves of this species is believed to be the reason why the herb has soothing, emollient qualities.

TRADITIONAL USES: Mallow has been eaten and used medicinally for thousands of years. In Costa Rica it is thought to stimulate lactation. It is also sold as an emollient and for use as an enema. According to Fetrow and Avila, mallow is used for irritations of the throat, bronchitis, laryngitis, tonsillitis, and hoarseness. It has also been used in Central America and the Caribbean to treat sores and wounds, as well as as an astringent.

AVAILABILITY AND DOSAGE: It is available as a dried leaf or flower. Fetrow and Avila report that the suggested dose is 5 grams daily of chopped, dried herb; an infusion may also be used.

CONTRAINDICATIONS: Fetrow and Avila recommend it not be used by pregnant or breast-feeding women.

SPECIAL PRECAUTIONS: Consult your physician before beginning any use of an ethnobotanical substance for medicinal purposes.

MEDICAL RESEARCH: None noted.

 Manaca

SCIENTIFIC NAME: *Brunfelsia uniflorus*
OTHER COMMON NAMES: Manacan, vegetable mercury
GROWING AREAS: Native to areas of the Amazon basin

PHYSICAL DESCRIPTION: An ornamental shrub, manaca produces a beautiful yellow-white flower. In his work on medicinal plants, James Duke recounts a legend that the plant's name is attributed to a beautiful girl of the Tupi Indians of Brazil.

TRADITIONAL USES: The Tupi use the plant in their medicinal and magical practices, according to Duke, who notes that the Indians once used a root extract of manaca as an arrow poison and that the scraped bark is considered a strong purgative. The common name vegetable mercury stems from the plant's use in traditional medicine for the treatment of syphilis. Based on his extensive travels in the Amazon area, botanist Richard Schultes reports that indigenous peoples use manaca as a treatment for rheumatism, as a diuretic, as an anti-inflammatory, to reduce fevers, and sometimes as an abortifacient. It has also been used as a hallucinogen, but with bad effects, Schultes writes.

AVAILABILITY AND DOSAGE: It is available as cut-and-sifted bark. Dosages vary.

CONTRAINDICATIONS: Since it is reported to have been used as an abortifacient, it should not be used by pregnant women.

SPECIAL PRECAUTIONS: Consult your physician before beginning any use of an ethnobotanical substance for medicinal purposes.

Manaca is reported to be toxic to children and pets and should be avoided.

MEDICAL RESEARCH: Laboratory tests in Brazil showed manaca to have anti-inflammatory properties. An extract of a related species, *Brunfelsia hopeana,* was shown in an experiment with rats to act as a central nervous system depressant and an anti-inflammatory. However, toxicological studies done in the United States of another species, *Brunfelsia calcyina*, determined that the consumption by dogs of this plant material was fatal, and researchers cautioned that the plant poses a significant hazard for small children. Duke says that even small doses of the alkaloid manacine, which is found in manaca, can lead to death due to respiratory paralysis in laboratory animals.

❧ Maracuja

SCIENTIFIC NAME: *Passiflora incarnata*

OTHER COMMON NAMES: Passionflower, maypop, passionaria, maracuya

GROWING AREAS: Native to Central and South America and parts of the southern United States; cultivated in Europe and North America

PHYSICAL DESCRIPTION: It is a climbing vine that can grow close to 30 feet long. Maracuja, or passionflower, as it is commonly called, has a three-lobed leaf that resembles a trident. Its flower is distinctive and has five stamens.

TRADITIONAL USES: Legend has it that following the conquest of the Incas by the Spaniards, a priest, looking for a divine sign that Spain's action was proper, discovered a flower on a vine in the Andes that symbolized the crucifixion of Christ. The flower's five stamens have come to symbolize the five wounds of Christ on the cross, and its three styles stand for the three nails used in the crucifixion.

After its discovery by the priest, passionflower was imported to Europe as a tea and was used as a sedative. In the United States it has been used as a sedative and to treat insomnia, anxiety, and panic. Experts also report that it is used to relax muscles and can relieve the discomfort of menstruation. By reducing anxiety, passionflower may also have other collateral effects on the body, such as lowering high blood pressure.

While passionflower was considered a sedative for many years in the United States, it was reported that the Food and Drug Administration removed it from the list of herbs generally considered as safe in 1978 because it was not proven effective as a sleeping aid. However, in Europe it is considered safe and useful in treating nervous restlessness.

AVAILABILITY AND DOSAGE: It is available as a dried herb, liquid extract, and tincture. Dosages vary. Some herbalists recommend dosages for tea ranging from 0.5 grams to 2.5 grams of the herb in boiling water up to three times daily. Commission E recommends 4 to 8 grams in a preparation. Herbal experts recommend a teaspoon of crushed leaves steeped in a cup of boiling water for about ten minutes to help with insomnia.

CONTRAINDICATIONS: It has been reported that in Norway a number of patients admitted to a hospital with altered states of consciousness had taken an insomnia remedy that was derived from passionflower. It was believed that the product may have interacted with other drugs to cause an intoxicating effect. Some experts also believe it is contraindicated for pregnant and breast-feeding women.

SPECIAL PRECAUTIONS: Consult your physician before beginning any use of an ethnobotanical substance for medicinal purposes.

Since passionflower appears to act on the central nervous system, it may interact with other depressants. It may also contain a uterine stimulant.

MEDICAL RESEARCH: A series of experiments with mice who received injections of passionflower extracts has shown that the plant contains chemicals that act as a central nervous system depressant. In one French study, mice showed reduced activity when treated with a water extract. In addition, the extract caused the mice to go to sleep when it followed a dose of phenobarbital. But the strength of the tranquilizer seems to depend on the solvent used to prepare the extract. For instance, when an extract was prepared with a water and alcohol agent, the mice appeared to show more activity, not less. Other studies with rodents show general sedative activity of the passionflower extract, including an instance when rats showed diminished activity when they were kept for a three-week period on oral doses of passionflower.

Mozote

SCIENTIFIC NAME: *Triumfetta semitriloba*

OTHER COMMON NAMES: Pega pega, burr bush, mozote de caballo

GROWING AREAS: Native to Central America, the Caribbean, and parts of South America

PHYSICAL DESCRIPTION: Mozote is a shrub that grows to a height of about 3 feet. Its leaves are generally three-lobed and toothed. It produces a yellow flower, and the undersides of the leaves are hairy.

TRADITIONAL USES: In Costa Rica mozote is used as a treatment for colds and diarrhea. According to Julia Morton, Mexicans use a decoction of the root for treating venereal disease, as well as kidney and liver problems, while a more astringent leaf decoction is used in Yucatán to treat hemorrhoids and leukorrhea.

AVAILABILITY AND DOSAGE: Available by mail order in the United States and Central America. No information available on dosage.

CONTRAINDICATIONS: Should be avoided by pregnant women.

SPECIAL PRECAUTIONS: Consult your physician before beginning any use of an ethnobotanical substance for medicinal purposes.

MEDICAL RESEARCH: None noted.

Mugwort

SCIENTIFIC NAME: *Artemisia vulgaris*

OTHER COMMON NAMES: Ajenjo, carline thistle (a related herb, *Artemisia absinthium*, is known in Mexican culture as ajenjo and also commonly known in English as wormwood, and is considered a more dangerous herb)

GROWING AREAS: Native to North America and China

PHYSICAL DESCRIPTION: It is an ornamental plant with lobed leaves, which grow in sets of two on the stem.

TRADITIONAL USES: Anglo-Saxons considered it a sacred

herb, and it is said by historians to have been used by Roman soldiers, who placed sprigs of the plant in their shoes to prevent foot problems during long marches. It is used in modern times as a treatment for dysmenorrhea, colic, diarrhea, constipation, and cramps. It is also considered an anthelmintic (a substance that destroys or causes the body to expel intestinal worms) and an emmenagogue. Russians reportedly have used it as an abortifacient and for bladder stones, and there are additional reports that it is useful for depression and neuroses.

AVAILABILITY AND DOSAGE: It is available as a dried leaf or root, as well as in a fluid extract and tincture. Herbalists recommend varying dosages, including up to 5 grams in a decoction for menstrual pain. Some experts recommend an infusion of up to 15 grams of the dried plant for such pain.

CONTRAINDICATIONS: Because it can cause uterine contractions, it should not be used by pregnant women. Breast-feeding women should not use it.

SPECIAL PRECAUTIONS: Consult your physician before beginning any use of an ethnobotanical substance for medicinal purposes.

Mugwort is believed to cause uterine contractions and may cause contact dermatitis, according to some experts. Avila and Fetrow caution that patients taking anticoagulants or with bleeding problems should not take mugwort. Duke reports that in large doses mugwort can be toxic and that a constituent element, thujone, can cause epileptic seizures. It may also cause dermatitis and allergic reaction in some people.

MEDICAL RESEARCH: None noted.

Muira Puama

SCIENTIFIC NAME: *Ptychopetalum olacoides*

OTHER COMMON NAMES: Potency wood, marapuama, marapama, potenzholz

GROWING AREAS: Native to the Amazon region, particularly Brazil

PHYSICAL DESCRIPTION: It is a bush that grows up to 15 feet in height and produces a small white flower that has a jasminelike fragrance, said Leslie Taylor.

TRADITIONAL USES: Based on his extensive travels and observations in South America, Richard Schultes reports that muira puama is used to treat neuromuscular problems, baldness, rheumatism, asthma, and gastrointestinal and cardiac problems. A bath of the root is used to treat paralysis. However, its major use is as an aphrodisiac tonic in the Amazon. James Duke also reports that the drug has a long history of use in Brazil as an aphrodisiac and nerve stimulant.

Commission E has noted that while muira puama is used to prevent sexual problems and as an aphrodisiac, its effectiveness has not been documented and that it is not approved for use. However, an extract of muira puama has been marketed in Europe under the names Herbal v-Y and Herbal v-X to treat impotency in men and sexual problems in women.

AVAILABILITY AND DOSAGE: It is available as a bark powder and as a concentrated liquid extract. Herbal formulas in tablet form were available in Europe in the late 1990s.

CONTRAINDICATIONS: Reported to be contraindicated for persons taking MAO inhibitors.

SPECIAL PRECAUTIONS: Consult your physician before beginning any use of an ethnobotanical substance for medicinal purposes. Muira puama should not be taken during pregnancy or lactation.

MEDICAL RESEARCH: Researchers in France are reported to have used herbal preparations from muira puama for over a decade with one hundred impotent male patients, over 60 percent of whom reported significant improvement in their sex lives after a month's use.

Nettle

SCIENTIFIC NAME: *Urtica dioica*

OTHER COMMON NAMES: Common nettle, big string nettle, stinging nettle

GROWING AREAS: Temperate regions of the world

PHYSICAL DESCRIPTION: It is a perennial bush that can grow up to 7 feet tall. Its leaves are triangular-shaped and edged with points. It produces a flower that ranges in color from white to yellow. Bristles on the leaves and stems can sting, hence the common name.

TRADITIONAL USES: The major interest in nettle today is in its use to treat benign prostatic hyperplasia (BPH), or enlarged prostate gland, a common condition for men over the age of fifty. It is used in combination with another herb, saw palmetto, for prostate health. But over the ages nettle has had a number of medicinal uses. Dioscorides listed it in his famous book of herbal remedies from the first century as a treatment for nosebleeds. The ancient Greeks used it to treat coughs and arthritis. It has a history of use as an astringent, to treat skin conditions, and as a remedy for baldness. It was also used to promote childbirth and stop uterine bleeding. It is used as a diuretic and as therapy for rheumatism and inflammations of the urinary tract.

AVAILABILITY AND DOSAGE: Nettle is available as a capsule and as an extract, powder, or tincture of the root and leaf. Dosages may vary and can range from a recommended intake of one capsule of 100 milligrams a day to a total of 300 milligrams. Teas can be made of up to 2 teaspoons per cup twice a day. Commission E recommends dosages between 8 and 10 grams of the herb and leaf daily and 4 to 6 grams of the root. It is also available as an element in herbal preparations.

CONTRAINDICATIONS: Commission E reported that no contraindications were known. However, some pharmacists report that nettle is contraindicated in pregnant women because it is a stimulant of uterine contractions. Breast-feeding women should also not use it.

SPECIAL PRECAUTIONS: Consult your physician before beginning any use of an ethnobotanical substance for medicinal purposes.

Internal use has been known to cause occasional gastrointestinal upset. The hairs on the plant contain chemicals that can cause severe skin irritation.

MEDICAL RESEARCH: Nettle does not appear to reduce the enlarged prostate gland in humans but rather increases the flow and volume of urine, according to the findings of Commission E. However, some research done in Germany has indicated that nettle inhibits prostatic hyperplasia in mice. In the German experiments, the prostate glands of mice were treated to create prostatic hyperplasia and five preparations of stinging nettle root extract, each prepared with a different method of liquid extraction, were tested. The experiment found that ethanol extracts and water extracts had the greatest effect on inhibiting the growth of the mice prostate glands. However, the researchers were unclear as to how the extracts worked. Another experiment, done in Japan on prostate tissue taken from a human patient suffering from an enlarged gland, suggested that steroids and other components in the stinging nettle roots inhibit prostate cell growth and metabolism.

Oregano

SCIENTIFIC NAME: *Lippia graveolens, Origanum vulgare*

OTHER COMMON NAMES: Oregano castillo, yerba dulce, wild marjoram

GROWING AREAS: *Lippia graveolens* grows in temperate and tropical areas.

PHYSICAL DESCRIPTION: *Lippia graveolens* is a shrub that grows up to 6 feet in height and has aromatic flowers.

TRADITIONAL USES: There are about forty different plants known by the name oregano. *Lippia graveolens* and related plants are known as a food seasoning. But oregano also has a long history of use as a medicinal plant. The Chinese are reported to have used it beginning in ancient times to treat fever, diarrhea, and vomiting. Among Mexicans, a species of oregano *(Monarda menthaefolia)* is listed in one survey as being among the top ten medicinal plants used in their culture to treat the symptoms of cold and flu, as well as coughs, sore throat, and congestion. Based upon fieldwork done in Belize,

Balick and Arvigo found that oregano is used as a tea to treat upper respiratory tract infections, induce menstruation, and, when taken a week after childbirth as a leaf decoction, to help a new mother expel a retained placenta. A boiled leaf solution is also said to be a good wash for wounds and burns.

AVAILABILITY AND DOSAGE: Oregano is widely available in supermarkets and food stores. The essential oil derived from the plant is also available, though herbalists caution that it should not be taken internally. For treating colds, teas made with boiling water using up to 3 teaspoons of herb or up to half a cup of fresh leaves as much as three times a day are recommended by some experts.

CONTRAINDICATIONS: Pregnant women should not use medicinal amounts of oregano, as it has a history of use as a uterine stimulant. Some experts say oregano can interfere with the absorption of iron.

SPECIAL PRECAUTIONS: Consult your physician before beginning any use of an ethnobotanical substance for medicinal purposes.

Experts caution that children under the age of two should not be given medicinal amounts of oregano. It may also produce allergic reactions and gastrointestinal discomfort.

MEDICAL RESEARCH: Oregano was found to inhibit the growth of eleven different microbes in one Australian study.

🌿 Papaya

SCIENTIFIC NAME: *Carica papaya*

OTHER COMMON NAMES: Paw paw, melon tree, put, papaya real

GROWING AREAS: Native to Mexico and Central America; cultivated in the Caribbean and Asia, as well as other tropical areas

PHYSICAL DESCRIPTION: Papaya is a tree with a thick trunk that can grow up to 25 feet high. Its leaves are lobed, can grow up to 2 feet across, and resemble those of an oak. The papaya tree produces a large (up to 11 pounds) oval-shaped fruit that hangs from the trunk; its yellowish pulp is sweet. A latex substance is obtained from its stem, leaves, and fruit.

TRADITIONAL USES: For centuries, people in the Caribbean knew of papaya's ability to tenderize meat, and the leaves are still used for that purpose today. This characteristic is attributed to a number of enzymes, notably papain, which are contained in the latex of the unripe papaya fruit and help to break down protein. In traditional medicine, papaya has been used to aid digestion, most certainly because papain acts similarly to human peptic acids. In Belize, the plant is used to help in the healing of wounds and infections, while the green fruit, when boiled and eaten, is said to aid in the purging of intestinal parasites, report Balick and Arvigo. They also report that women have used roasted and ground papaya seeds in a formula for contraception.

AVAILABILITY AND DOSAGE: Papaya fruit is readily available in the United States in food and fruit stores. Papaya enzyme is also available in tablet form. Doses may vary, although some herbalists recommend using a tea made from 1 or 2 teaspoons of dried papaya leaf before meals as an aid to digestion.

CONTRAINDICATIONS: Pregnant women should not use medicinal amounts of papaya, as it has a history of use as a uterine stimulant. Breast-feeding women should also not use it.

SPECIAL PRECAUTIONS: Consult your physician before beginning any use of an ethnobotanical substance for medicinal purposes.

Excessive use of papaya may cause gastric upset, allergic reaction, and possibly perforation of the esophagus, according to experts. It may also act as a purge if too much is taken. Ingestion by dogs of papain has been linked to birth defects. An extract of the fruit has been shown to affect human cardiac activity.

MEDICAL RESEARCH: According to Balick and Arvigo, a number of studies have been done that show papaya to have antibacterial and antifungal activity. They also reported that a study from 1947 showed that a water extract of the papaya fruit worked as a human cardiac depressant. Human clinical trials indicate that papaya can treat inflammation from surgery or accident and that it can be used to reduce postoperative edema in cases of head and neck surgery, write Fetrow and Avila.

Pau d'Arco

SCIENTIFIC NAME: *Tabebuia impetiginosa*
OTHER COMMON NAMES: Lapachol, lapacho, trumpet bush

GROWING AREAS: Native to South and Central America

PHYSICAL DESCRIPTION: It is a large flowering evergreen tree that can grow up to 15 feet high. The tree produces a large pink flower. The tree's durable wood has made it a target of loggers in the Amazon area, according to concerned environmentalists. There has also been concern raised over the harvesting of the tree's inner bark to produce folk medicine.

TRADITIONAL USES: Pau d'arco's history as a medicinal plant has been controversial. In folk medicine, lapachol is obtained from the inner bark of the tree and has been used in Latin America for the treatment of colds, flu, arthritis, rheumatism, syphilis, and cancer. It also has been used to treat disorders of the immune system such as psoriasis. Because of pau d'arco's traditional use to treat cancer in some cultures, it has received a great deal of attention and publicity as a possible cure. But despite great fanfare, testing of the extracts from the plant have, according to a number of experts and government officials, not supported the use of lapachol as a treatment for cancer. AIDS patients have also turned to pau d'arco as an alternative treatment, most likely because it has a reputation as a remedy for immune system problems.

AVAILABILITY AND DOSAGE: Pau d'arco is available in capsules, tablets, extracts, and teas. The bark is sold as a powder. Dosages may vary and run from 1 to 4 capsules a day for a week. Some suppliers recommend 300 milligrams of powdered bark three times a day. A tea is also made by boiling the bark in water for eight to ten minutes.

CONTRAINDICATIONS: Pau d'arco contains substances that researchers believe can cause problems with coagulation, which makes use of the plant questionable for people suffering from coagulation disorders or taking anticoagulants. Experts also say pregnant and breast-feeding women should avoid the herb.

SPECIAL PRECAUTIONS: Consult your physician before beginning any use of an ethnobotanical substance for medicinal purposes.

Certain substances in pau d'arco present a danger of toxicity in humans. Fetrow and Avila recommend that pau d'arco not be used because of the problem of toxicity.

MEDICAL RESEARCH: During the 1960s, after it gained a reputation as a folk treatment for cancer, lapachol was put into clinical trials by the National Cancer Institute. However, in 1974 it was reportedly dropped by the NCI after failing to produce significant results that outweighed its serious side effects. The negative experience of the NCI apparently did not forestall others from experimenting with lapachol as a cancer therapy, and there have been reports of trials in other countries that have shown beneficial results.

While cancer experiments in the United States did not go well, lapachol seemed to fare better with experiments aimed at testing its usefulness as an antipsoriatic and anti-inflammatory agent. In an experiment in Brazil, lapachol was found to have significant anti-inflammatory action, diminishing swelling in rodents by as much as 85 percent, depending on the dosage. Results of another experiment published in 1999 showed that lapachol compounds stopped the growth of human keratinocytes, the cells involved in psoriasis.

🌿 Pedra Hume Caa

SCIENTIFIC NAME: *Myrcia salicifolia*

OTHER COMMON NAMES: Insulina vegetal

GROWING AREAS: Native to South America and the West Indies

PHYSICAL DESCRIPTION: *Myrcia salicifolia* is a shrub with small green leaves and large orange-red flowers, said Leslie Taylor.

TRADITIONAL USES: In the Amazon, researchers found it to be used by Indians as a treatment for severe diarrhea and as an astringent and emetic. It has also been used to treat diabetes.

AVAILABILITY AND DOSAGE: It is available in the United States as cut-and-sifted leaf. Dosages vary. Herbalists recommend a half cup of the leaf infusion two or three times a day.

CONTRAINDICATIONS: Diabetics run the risk of hypoglycemia.

SPECIAL PRECAUTIONS: Consult your physician before beginning any use of an ethnobotanical substance for medicinal purposes.

MEDICAL RESEARCH: Research has shown that it has an inhibiting effect on serum glucose levels in diabetic rodents. One experiment involving the feeding of rats for three weeks with an extract of *Myrcia uniflora* improved metabolism of glucose compounds. However, another study detected no beneficial effect.

🌿 Periwinkle

SCIENTIFIC NAME: *Catharanthus roseus*

OTHER COMMON NAMES: Rosy periwinkle, vinca rosea, chata

GROWING AREAS: Native to Madagascar; cultivated in numerous other places

PHYSICAL DESCRIPTION: It is an herb that grows to a height of about 3 feet. Its leaves are green and shiny, and it produces a pink flower.

TRADITIONAL USES: The periwinkle is one of the best examples of a plant that has become a prime source of medicine for humans, serving as the basis for drugs to combat Hodgkin's disease and childhood leukemia. While originating in Madagascar, it was brought to Europe in the eighteenth century and spread from there, often being used as an ornamental plant. Before it began to be used as a source of modern drugs, periwinkle had a long history as a treatment for tumors, asthma, and diabetes and for use as an astringent, diuretic, and to increase menstrual flow. In parts of Central America and the Caribbean, the root and leaf are used to treat diabetes.

AVAILABILITY AND DOSAGE: It is available in the form of a powder. Dosages vary. Herbalists recommend using a teaspoon of dried herb to make an infusion that can be consumed up to three times a day. Two medicines derived from periwinkle, vinblastine for Hodgkin's disease and vincristine for childhood leukemia, are used by doctors as part of therapeutic regimes.

CONTRAINDICATIONS: See "Special Precautions."

SPECIAL PRECAUTIONS: Consult your physician before

beginning any use of an ethnobotanical substance for medicinal purposes.

Commission E reports that periwinkle has proved to be destructive to blood components in animal experiments. Because most of its claimed uses have not been documented, Commission E states that the use of periwinkle is not justified.

MEDICAL RESEARCH: Periwinkle has been extensively studied by scientists, who have identified over seventy alkaloids from the plant parts, including vincristine and vinblastine. The investigation of periwinkle began in the 1950s, when the National Cancer Institute began a program of screening plant chemicals for possible use against leukemia. Some pharmaceutical companies involved in the study expanded the search and found anti-cancer activity in a number of the alkaloids. Vinblastine was isolated in 1961 and approved for the treatment of Hodgkin's disease and testicular and breast cancer. Two years later vincristine was licensed for use against childhood leukemia. "Long term, disease-free survivals have been observed in the treatment of various lymphomas and leukemias, bladder cancer, and testicular cancer, while significant palliative benefits have been seen in patients with breast cancer, melanoma, and small-cell lung cancer," write Gordon M. Cragg and Michael R. Boyd of the NCI.

🌿 Picao Preto

SCIENTIFIC NAME: *Bidens pilosa*

OTHER COMMON NAMES: Black Jack, Spanish nettle, mozote

GROWING AREAS: Native to South America, Africa, and the Caribbean

PHYSICAL DESCRIPTION: *Bidens pilosa* is a small annual herb that grows to a height of about 3 feet. It has a small yellow flower.

TRADITIONAL USES: It is reported to be used in the Peruvian Amazon for a number of ailments, including angina, dysentery, and worms. It is also used in Peru as a diuretic and anti-inflammatory, as well as to speed childbirth and as a treatment for hepatitis, according to Leslie Taylor.

AVAILABILITY AND DOSAGE: It is available in the United States as a powder. Dosages vary. Herbalists recommend a half cup of the decoction three times a day.

CONTRAINDICATIONS: Since it is reported to be used as a uterine stimulant, it should be avoided by pregnant women.

SPECIAL PRECAUTIONS: Consult your physician before beginning any use of an ethnobotanical substance for medicinal purposes.

Brazilian researchers have said that the use of *Bidens pilosa* must await clarification of the plant's toxicity because a link with esophageal cancer has been suggested.

MEDICAL RESEARCH: *Bidens pilosa* was among fifty-four plant extracts tested in an experiment of anti-bacterial activity in South Africa. Five types of bacteria were used in the study, including *E. coli* and two types of staphylococcus. The bacteria were placed in sterile petri dishes, the extracts were then introduced, and the antibacterial activity was determined by the size of the zone of inhibition or clear space where the organism did not grow. The *Bidens pilosa* extract was found to have some of the highest antibacterial activity against the staphylococcus strains, but not the *E. coli*. The results tended to support the traditional medicinal uses of the plant, the researchers concluded.

Quinine Bark

SCIENTIFIC NAME: *Cinchona officinalis*

OTHER COMMON NAMES: Cinchona, fever tree, cinchona bark

GROWING AREAS: Native to South America, primarily in the area of the Peruvian Amazon basin; also cultivated in other areas of the region and in Java and India

PHYSICAL DESCRIPTION: Cinchona is an evergreen that can reach a height of over 75 feet. It has a deep reddish bark and produces yellow-and-white flowers. There are about forty related tree species.

TRADITIONAL USES: For many centuries, cinchona has been used by the indigenous peoples of Peru, including the Incas, for malaria, digestive problems, and fever. It is known to stimulate secretion of saliva and digestive juices. Western contact with cinchona arose during the Spanish conquest of the Americas. Some legends hold that a sick Spanish soldier drank from a pool of water into which a cinchona tree had fallen, while another story holds that the wife of the viceroy of Peru was cured by the bark and reported to Europe about the marvels of cinchona. Whatever the truth may be, cinchona became widely accepted in the West as a cure for malaria, which had been a problem in European cities at one time. In 1820, French chemists Joseph Caventou and Joseph Pelletier identified and isolated the alkaloid quinine from cinchona bark. The need for quinine, an agent effective against the mosquito-transmitted protozoan that causes malaria, required a substantial export trade from South America, which led to a monopoly. Finally the monopoly was broken when cinchona seeds were cultivated in Dutch Java, which came to dominate the world trade in cinchona.

During World War II American officials were almost without any source of quinine because of Japanese conquests in the Far East. U.S. officials then turned to the forests of South America to get cinchona bark so that quinine could be extracted. After the war, new antimalarial drugs began to be manufactured and the demand for cinchona dropped off, although it remained useful in treating heart arrhythmias and had a long-standing use as a flavoring agent. However, the appearance of malaria parasites resistant to the new drugs has renewed interest in quinine as a treatment.

AVAILABILITY AND DOSAGE: It is available in the United States as an herb powder made from bark. Commission E recommends 1 to 3 grams of the dried bark; 0.6 to 3 grams of cinchona liquid extract (4 to 5 percent total alkaloids); 0.15 to 0.6 grams of cinchona extract (15 to 20 percent total alkaloids). Herbalists recommend that a half cup of the bark decoction can be taken one to three times daily.

CONTRAINDICATIONS: Herbalists warn that cinchona is not to be taken by pregnant or breast-feeding women. Persons with allergies to cinchona alkaloids are also cautioned about its use. Commission E states that it may increase the effect of anticoagulants.

SPECIAL PRECAUTIONS: Consult your physician before beginning any use of an ethnobotanical substance for medicinal purposes.

Herbalists caution that it should be used only under medical supervision. Cinchona is reputed to be toxic when used excessively and can lead to nausea, deafness, and other physical problems. Contact dermatitis and asthma are sometimes reported to have stricken workers in factories where cinchona bark was ground.

MEDICAL RESEARCH: The scientific literature is filled with information about the efficacy of cinchona in the treatment of malaria and arrhythmia. A survey of medicinal plants also shows that cinchona is used as an antiepileptic treatment.

❧ Rhatany

SCIENTIFIC NAME: *Krameria triandra*

OTHER COMMON NAMES: Raiz para, mapato, Peruvian rhatany, pumacuchu

GROWING AREAS: Western slopes of the Andes in Peru, Ecuador, and Bolivia, at altitudes of up to 10,000 feet

PHYSICAL DESCRIPTION: Rhatany is an evergreen shrub that grows about 3 feet in height and produces a large red flower. Its root, the part that is used medicinally, is deep.

TRADITIONAL USES: The major traditional use of rhatany is as an astringent and for gastrointestinal problems. It is also reported to be used by indigenous peoples as a tooth preservative. Herbalists say it is useful as a mouthwash and to treat sore throat and canker sores. Commission E reports that it is used as a topical treatment for inflammations on the oral and pharyngeal mucosae. The primary active ingredients are tannins.

AVAILABILITY AND DOSAGE: Commission E recommends about 1 gram of powdered root in a cup of water as a decoction or 5 to 10 drops of rhatany tincture in a glass of water three times a day.

CONTRAINDICATIONS: Fetrow and Avila report that rhatany is contraindicated for persons sensitive to substances in the plant.

SPECIAL PRECAUTIONS: Consult your physician before beginning any use of an ethnobotanical substance for medicinal purposes.

Fetrow and Avila warn that products containing tannic acid are generally considered unsafe and ineffective and that frequent use can compromise the mucous membranes so that toxicity results. Commission E says that allergic reactions of the mucous membranes may occur in rare cases.

MEDICAL RESEARCH: None noted.

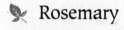 Rosemary

SCIENTIFIC NAME: *Rosemarinus officinalis*
OTHER COMMON NAMES: Romero, compass plant, old man

GROWING AREAS: Native to southern Europe; grows in
the United States, Mexico, Central America, and South
America

PHYSICAL DESCRIPTION: Rosemary is a perennial evergreen shrub that is very aromatic and grows from 3 to
7 feet in height. It has narrow green leaves resembling
pine needles.

TRADITIONAL USES: A useful cooking herb, rosemary is
long on legend and lore. It was considered to enhance
memory in ancient times, so much so that students are
said to have burned it at home before exams or worn it
in garlands. It was used to preserve meats in the days
before refrigeration, and it became a symbol of remembrance during funerals. In *Hamlet*, Ophelia remarks to
the king, "There's rosemary, that's for remembrance.
Pray you, love, remember." In European folklore it was
believed to stave off bad dreams and was a symbol of
love. Legend has it that Queen Elizabeth of Hungary in
the thirteenth century was cured of the pain of rheumatism after her limbs were bathed in a wine decoction
containing rosemary.

Medicinally, rosemary has been used as an astringent, anti-inflammatory, and antiseptic, as well as an
abortifacient, emmenagogue, and tonic. In parts of
Central America rosemary has been used for nervous
disorders, to cleanse wounds and skin ulcers, to relieve
headaches, and for washing hair. A poll of Mexicans
found rosemary to be among the top herbs they listed as
being used medicinally, largely for menstrual and digestive problems.

AVAILABILITY AND DOSAGE: Rosemary is found in herb

form in supermarkets and other food stores. It is also available as a tea or essential oil. Some herbalists recommend that the essential oil be used externally or in a diffuser to permeate the atmosphere. Herbalists recommend that a tea can be made from up to 4 grams of leaf and taken as often as three times a day.

CONTRAINDICATIONS: Rosemary should not be taken in medicinal quantities by pregnant or breast-feeding women.

SPECIAL PRECAUTIONS: Consult your physician before beginning any use of an ethnobotanical substance for medicinal purposes.

While the undiluted essential oil has a history of being taken internally, a number of experts believe it should not be consumed because it can lead to stomach or other gastrointestinal problems. German experts, however, have approved rosemary for internal use for indigestion and rheumatism.

MEDICAL RESEARCH: Essential oil of rosemary was noted by European researchers as being among a group of powerful convulsants.

🌿 Rue

SCIENTIFIC NAME: *Ruta graveolens*

OTHER COMMON NAMES: Ruda, ruta, garden rue, German rue

GROWING AREAS: Native to Europe; widely grown in Latin America

PHYSICAL DESCRIPTION: Rue is a small, erect bush that

grows to a height of about 3 feet. The shoots of the plant are pale green and appear covered in oil glands. It produces small yellow flowers, and its fruit contains rutin, the volatile oil that gives it a bitter taste.

TRADITIONAL USES: In ancient times, rue was considered a major remedy. It is mentioned more than eighty times by Pliny, but its reputation has lessened because it can be toxic. Still, it is reportedly used in a number of cultures as a beverage, and it is used in Costa Rica as an antispasmodic, emmenagogue, abortifacient, emetic, disinfectant, diuretic, and as a treatment for epilepsy and worms. It is also used to speed labor in childbirth. Rue water is used as an insecticide and flea repellent. As a liniment, it is used on sore muscles.

Hispanics in the United States have reported using rue to treat *empacho* and *mal ojo*. *Curanderos* use rue as part of their *limpias*, or ritual spiritual cleansings. It is sometimes worn in amulets.

AVAILABILITY AND DOSAGE: It is available through mail order and as a dried herb and liquid extract. Dosages vary.

CONTRAINDICATIONS: Since rue causes abortions and uterine contractions and can act as an emmenagogue, it should not be used by pregnant women. Breast-feeding women should also not use it.

SPECIAL PRECAUTIONS: Consult your physician before beginning any use of an ethnobotanical substance for medicinal purposes.

Despite its wide use, rue is one of the more dangerous plants used medicinally. It is known to be an abortifacient and to cause skin irritation. It has also been known to cause severe stomach problems and vomiting and, according to Balick, has been reported in some cases to be fatal to the mother when used to cause an abortion. Given the various problems associated with it, rue should be avoided.

MEDICAL RESEARCH: Rue has been shown in animal experiments to act as an anticonvulsant, and extracts of it displayed antibacterial and antituberculosis activity in laboratory experiments, according to Balick and Arvigo. In other experiments, chloroform extracts of the root, stem, and leaf of the plant showed significant antifertility activity in rats.

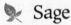 Sage

SCIENTIFIC NAME: *Salvia officinalis*

OTHER COMMON NAMES: Garden sage, salvia, meadow sage, salvia virgen

GROWING AREAS: Native to southern Europe; widely cultivated

PHYSICAL DESCRIPTION: Sage is a perennial evergreen shrub that grows about 3 feet high. Its leaves are oval, green, and velvety. Its flowers, which bloom in the summer, run from white to purple.

TRADITIONAL USES: Like many medicinal herbs, sage is widely used in cooking. But sage also has a long reputation for treating a number of medical conditions, and its genus name, *Salvia*, derives from the Latin, meaning "to cure." Historians also note that a medieval saying by Italian medical students asserted, "Why should a man die who grows sage in his garden?" According to herb expert Michael Castleman, sage was used by the ancient

Greeks and Romans as a meat preservative, as a memory enhancer, to treat problems such as epilepsy and snakebite, and to promote menstrual flow.

In more modern times, sage has been used as an antiseptic and astringent, a digestive tonic, an antiperspirant, and a method for controlling irregular menstruation and menopausal problems. A preparation of sage is used as a gargle for sore throat, mouth ulcers, sore gums, and tonsillitis. In Costa Rica, sage is used for wounds, arthritis, asthma, and problems with the prostate gland. It is also a commonly used herb among Mexicans. In Europe it has been used to lower blood sugar in diabetics.

AVAILABILITY AND DOSAGE: Dried leaves are available in food stores and in *botánicas* for further home preparation. Sage is also available through suppliers as a liquid extract. The dosages vary according to the herbalist. For a gargle, a weak infusion is recommended, using from one to four leaves. For menstruation problems, a tincture of up to 4 milliliters of leaf extract has been recommended by some experts. Fresh sage leaf is also applied directly to stings or bites as a treatment.

CONTRAINDICATIONS: Use of sage should be avoided by pregnant women because of the herb's reputation for causing abortions. Diabetic patients also have to use sage cautiously because of its ability to lower blood sugar. Fetrow and Avila recommend that it be used carefully by persons already receiving anticonvulsants.

SPECIAL PRECAUTIONS: Consult your physician before beginning any use of an ethnobotanical substance for medicinal purposes.

While it has a long history as a medicinal herb, sage is viewed with caution by some doctors, pharmacists, and herbalists. In their professional handbook on alternative medicines, Fetrow and Avila advise that sage can interact with anticonvulsants, disulfiram, insulin, and other diabetic therapies. Herb expert Michael Castleman cautions that sage oil is toxic and should not be ingested. But he also notes that one toxic chemical contained in sage, thujone, while causing convulsions, is mostly eliminated by the heat of infusion preparation using plant leaves.

MEDICAL RESEARCH: None noted.

 Sarsaparilla

SCIENTIFIC NAME: *Smilax officinalis*

OTHER COMMON NAMES: Cuculmeca, zazaparilla, brown sarsaparilla

GROWING AREAS: Native to Central America and Colombia

PHYSICAL DESCRIPTION: Sarsaparilla is a woody vine that can grow to a length of about 15 feet. It has tendrils that help it climb, ovate (egg-shaped) leaves, and green flowers. Its root is narrow and very long and is used for medicinal purposes.

TRADITIONAL USES: The plant was brought from the New World to Spain, along with China root *(Smilax china)*, with great fanfare in the sixteenth century as a cure for syphilis after it had been used with some success in the Caribbean. It was listed in Nicholas Monardes's book *Joyful Newes out of the Newe Founde Worlde* as a wonderful medicinal plant of that time. However, its usefulness as a cure for venereal disease dropped off, although it continued to be used for that purpose well into the nineteenth century. It became a flavoring agent for root beer but has been replaced by artificial ingredients.

In traditional medicine, sarsaparilla has been used as a so-called blood purifier, as an anti-inflammatory, and as a cleansing agent. It is commonly used to treat psoriasis and eczema. It has steroid components and for that reason is reported to have been used by athletes as a performance-boosting medicine, as well as a possible treatment for impotence. It does not, however, contain testosterone, as some popularly believed. In Costa Rica it is used as a cold remedy and a tonic for boosting immunity, and in Jamaica it is used as a diuretic. Commission E reported that it is used for rheumatic complaints, for kidney diseases, and as a diuretic and diaphoretic.

AVAILABILITY AND DOSAGE: Sarsaparilla is available in powdered form as a tea or tablet and also as a liquid. For psoriasis, some experts recommend taking 1 to 4 grams of dried root or up to 30 milliliters of concentrated sarsaparilla compound as a decoction. A couple of teaspoons of powdered root as a decoction are also recommended as a diuretic.

CONTRAINDICATIONS: Pregnant or breast-feeding women should not use sarsaparilla. It is also contraindicated if an individual is taking digitalis or bismuth.

SPECIAL PRECAUTIONS: Consult your physician before beginning any use of an ethnobotanical substance for medicinal purposes.

Sarsaparilla is considered by the Food and Drug Administration as safe for use as a flavoring agent. However, Commission E labels it as a medicinal plant whose use is unapproved. The commission cautions that sarsaparilla can lead to gastric upset and temporary kidney impairment. Sarsaparilla may also affect the action of other herbs taken with it, and the commission cautions that it may also interact with digitalis and bismuth. Other experts say it can lead to nausea or kidney damage.

MEDICAL RESEARCH: Medical research into sarsaparilla, given its long history of use as a medicinal plant, is rather modest. One study from the 1940s found that psoriasis patients treated with sarsaparilla showed improvement. However, that study has been criticized because of its design. Sarsaparilla has shown anti-inflammatory activity in rodents. There have been reports of tests in China showing that up to 90 percent of acute cases of syphilis were effectively treated with sarsaparilla.

Sour Cane

SCIENTIFIC NAME: *Costus spicatus*

OTHER COMMON NAMES: Cana agria, canita agria, cana amarga

GROWING AREAS: Native to an area from Mexico to Brazil

PHYSICAL DESCRIPTION: A tall perennial plant with thin, fleshy stems. The leaves are egg-shaped and pointed at the tip with brown hairs on the edges.

TRADITIONAL USES: Sour cane contains a bitter-tasting sap that is obtained from the plant by crushing it. It is used in Central America for a variety of ailments. In Costa Rica it is used for muscle pain and kidney and urinary function, and is sold widely by herb vendors as a fresh item. In the West Indies, the plant decoction is taken to relieve flatulence and rheumatism, and in Trinidad it is used to relieve the urinary burning that accompanies venereal disease, according to Julia Morton. She also noted that some Brazilians drink the plant juice with sugar and water as a hot-weather beverage.

AVAILABILITY AND DOSAGE: Available by mail order. No information available on dosage.

CONTRAINDICATIONS: None noted.

SPECIAL PRECAUTIONS: Consult your physician before beginning any use of an ethnobotanical substance for medicinal purposes.

MEDICAL RESEARCH: None noted.

Thyme

SCIENTIFIC NAME: *Thymus vulgaris*

OTHER COMMON NAMES: Tomillo, mother of thyme, garden thyme

GROWING AREAS: Native to southern Europe; cultivated around the world

PHYSICAL DESCRIPTION: It is an aromatic shrub with woody stems, small leaves, and pink flowers.

TRADITIONAL USES: Thyme is another example of a plant that has long been used for both cooking and medicinal purposes. Pliny said it was useful as a treatment for headaches and snakebite, possibly because of the way the plant's stem resembles a serpent. In ancient times it was used as a cough remedy, to treat gastrointestinal problems, and to treat intestinal worms. During medieval times, women gave their knights scarves embroidered with sprigs of thyme as a symbol of bravery.

Herbalists from that period said thyme induced child-birth. By the eighteenth century, thyme's antiseptic properties were known, and its oil, known as thymol, was extracted and made available. It was used widely as an antiseptic up to World War I, when shortages of thymol developed. It gradually came to be replaced by other antiseptics.

Herbalists use thyme as an antiseptic, expectorant, massage oil, chest rub, and antibiotic. In Costa Rica the herb is used to combat intestinal worms and to treat warts, diarrhea, toothache, whooping cough, scabies, and flatulence. It is also considered a powerful strengthener of the lungs. Thymol is a key ingredient in Listerine, a popular mouthwash.

AVAILABILITY AND DOSAGE: Thyme is available in many supermarkets and health food stores. It is also available as a liquid extract and can also be purchased as a dried plant in *botánicas*. Thyme can be applied directly to the skin to relieve insect bites and help rheumatic pain. Infusions of up to 2 grams of dried herb can be used for tea. An infusion can also be used for a gargle. A dilution of essential oil of thyme can be used on skin for certain conditions.

CONTRAINDICATIONS: Since it has a history of use as a uterine stimulant, it should not be used by pregnant women. Fetrow and Avila caution that it should not be used by persons with a history of gastritis and intestinal disorders, nor by those allergic to plants such as grass, nor by those with enterocolitis or cardiac insufficiency.

SPECIAL PRECAUTIONS: Consult your physician before beginning any use of an ethnobotanical substance for medicinal purposes.

Pure thymol should not be taken internally, since even small amounts can be toxic. Thyme may cause allergic reactions in some persons.

MEDICAL RESEARCH: Thyme has been reported as exhibiting antifungal activity and showing spasmolytic action in animal tests.

❧ Witch Hazel

SCIENTIFIC NAME: *Hamamelis virginiana*

OTHER COMMON NAMES: Agua maravilla, winter bloom, spotted alder

GROWING AREAS: Native to the eastern United States

PHYSICAL DESCRIPTION: A perennial shrub that sheds its leaves in the fall, *Hamamelis virginiana* sends up a number of twisting stems that end in branches containing oval leaves. The plant's seed pods burst open with an audible popping sound and propel two black seeds several yards. The plant produces yellow flowers.

TRADITIONAL USES: Witch hazel is the extract prepared from the twigs of *Hamamelis virginiana* through a distillation process. It was used by Native Americans before the colonists arrived, and the settlers soon learned of witch hazel's astringent qualities. The name *witch hazel* is thought to derive from either the use of the plant's wood to make brooms or else the popping sound made by the seed pods, perhaps thought to be a hint of some occult power. In any case, a decoction of the plant became widely used as an astringent and antiseptic in the United States during the nineteenth century. It was then that controversy erupted following the commercial use of distillation to make extracts of witch hazel. According to author and herbal expert Michael Castleman, some critics contend that distillation removes many of the astringent tannins, leaving water that is of little medicinal value. Castleman has noted that while herbalists recommend that only a decoction of witch hazel be used, the commercially prepared liquid has properties that are reportedly antiseptic, anti-inflammatory, astringent, and anesthetic.

In Puerto Rican communities, a witch hazel compound known as agua maravilla is sometimes reported to be used as a therapy for asthma. The mixture, containing juice of aloe vera, honey, garlic, onion, and other substances, is ingested.

AVAILABILITY AND DOSAGE: Witch hazel is readily available in the United States in most pharmacies, supermarkets, and *botánicas*. It is also present in hemorrhoid preparations. Agua maravilla is available in *botánicas*. Herbalists recommend using up to 2 grams of dried leaves or bark to make a tea to use as a gargle. For an astringent decoction, a similar amount can be used per cup of boiling water. For external topical use, consult the directions on the product.

CONTRAINDICATIONS: Pregnant and breast-feeding women should avoid using it internally.

SPECIAL PRECAUTIONS: Consult your physician before beginning any use of an ethnobotanical substance for medicinal purposes.

There is the risk of nausea and vomiting if large amounts are ingested. Skin irritation may also result from topical use.

MEDICAL RESEARCH: None noted.

Wormwood

SCIENTIFIC NAME: *Artemisia absinthium*

OTHER COMMON NAMES: Artemisia, absinthe, ajenjo, estafiate

GROWING AREAS: Native to Europe; grows in the eastern United States

PHYSICAL DESCRIPTION: Wormwood is a perennial that has grayish-green stems. It can grow to a height of 4 feet, and its leaves, which are in blunt segments, have silvery hairs on both sides and resemble feathers.

TRADITIONAL USES: Beginning in the late eighteenth century, wormwood was used to give a popular liqueur called absinthe its bitter flavor. But within that alcoholic mix lurked a great danger. Thujone, a volatile oil within the plant, is believed to have a narcotic effect and is reported to have been responsible for hallucinations, psychosis, and possible brain damage, a syndrome labeled "absinthism." The great painter Vincent van Gogh was reported to have been a habitual user of absinthe, and experts believe the heavy use of yellow in his art may have resulted from thujone-caused brain damage. After much controversy, the drink was banned in France in the early twentieth century.

Herbalists report that wormwood is useful for expelling intestinal worms and stimulating the gastrointestinal tract and uterus. It is also reported to work as an anti-inflammatory. It is a Hispanic folk remedy for diarrhea, arthritis, gout, and late menstrual periods. In one survey of Mexicans and Mexican-Americans it was found to be one of the top ten herbal remedies used in households. In Central America it is used to treat rheumatism and neuralgia and for healing and toning the liver.

AVAILABILITY AND DOSAGE: Wormwood is available as a dried herb. It is used in infusions and decoctions. Tinctures and extracts are also sold. Experts say preparation by infusion usually requires using about ½ teaspoon; a decoction, up to 2 teaspoons in boiling water. Other dosages may vary.

CONTRAINDICATIONS: Should not be taken by pregnant or breast-feeding women.

SPECIAL PRECAUTIONS: Consult your physician before beginning any use of an ethnobotanical substance for medicinal purposes.

Because of the drug's thujone content, some experts warn that its administration can cause severe gastrointestinal distress, such as vomiting and cramps, and nervous system problems. They recommend against continuous use. Other experts believe the drug should not be used at home at all because of its history of problems.

MEDICAL RESEARCH: None noted.

Sources and Bibliography

BOOKS

Arvigo, Rosita, and Michael Balick, *Rainforest Remedies: One Hundred Healing Herbs of Belize* (2nd ed.). Twin Lakes, WI: Lotus Press, 1998.

Avila, Elena, with Joy Parker, *Woman Who Glows in the Dark.* New York: Jeremy P. Tarcher/Putnam, 1999.

Balick, Michael, and Paul Cox, *Plants, People, and Culture: The Science of Ethnobotany.* New York: Scientific American Library, 1999.

Balick, Michael, Elaine Elisabetsky, and Sarah A. Laird, eds., *Medicinal Resources of the Tropical Forest: Biodiversity and Its Importance to Human Health.* New York: Columbia University Press, 1996.

Bisset, Norman Grainger, ed., *Herbal Drugs and Phytopharmaceuticals.* Stuttgart: Medpharm Scientific Publishing, 1994.

Blumenthal, Mark, et al., eds., *The Complete German Commission E Monographs: Therapeutic Guide to Herbal Medicines.* Austin, TX: American Botanical Council, 1998.

Boettcher, Helmuth M., *Wonder Drugs: A History of Antibi-*

otics. Philadelphia and New York: J.B. Lippincott Co., 1963.

Castleman, Michael, *The Healing Herbs: The Ultimate Guide to the Curative Power of Nature's Medicines*. New York: Bantam Books, 1995.

Chevallier, Andrew, *The Encyclopedia of Medicinal Plants*. New York: D.K. Publishers Inc., 1996.

Coe, Michael D., *The Maya* (6th ed.). New York: Thames and Hudson, Inc., 1999.

Davidow, Joie, *Infusions of Healing: A Treasury of Mexican-American Herbal Remedies*. New York: Simon and Schuster, 1999.

Duke, James A., *CRC Handbook of Medicinal Herbs*. Boca Raton, FL: CRC Press, Inc., 1985.

Fetrow, Charles W., and Juan R. Avila, *Professional's Handbook of Complementary and Alternative Medicines*. Springhouse: Springhouse Corp., 1999.

Fleming, Thomas, et al., eds., *PDR for Herbal Medicines*. Montvale: Medical Economics Company, 1998.

Foster, Steven, and James A. Duke, *A Field Guide to Medicinal Plants*. Boston: Houghton Mifflin Company, 1990.

González-Wippler, Migene, *Santería: African Magic in Latin America* (2nd ed.). Plainview: Original Publications, 1992.

Griffin, Judy, *Mother Nature's Herbal*. St. Paul: Llewellyn Publications, 1997.

Griggs, Barbara, *Green Pharmacy: A History of Herbal Medicine*. New York: The Viking Press, 1981.

Joyce, Christopher, *Earthly Goods: Medicine Hunting in the Rainforests*. Boston and New York: Little, Brown and Company, 1994.

Kessler, David, M.D., *The Doctor's Complete Guide to*

Healing Herbs. New York: The Berkeley Publishing Group, 1996.

Mejia Ramirez, Jaime, *Some Medicinal Plants of Costa Rica.* Alajuela, Costa Rica: Imprenta y Lithografia Publicrex, 1995.

Meza, Elsa N., ed., *Desarrollando Nuestra Diversidad Biocultural: "Sangre de Grado" y el Reto de su Produccion Sustentable en el Peru.* Lima: Universidad Nacional Mayor de San Marcos Fondo Editorial, 1999.

Morley, Sylvanus G., and George W. Brainerd, *The Ancient Maya* (3rd ed.). Stanford: Stanford University Press, 1957.

Morton, Julia F., *The Atlas of Medicinal Plants of Middle America, Bahamas to Yucatan.* Springfield: Charles C. Thomas, 1981.

Murray, Michael T., *The Healing Power of Herbs* (2nd ed.). Rocklin, CA: Prima Publishing, 1995.

Ody, Penelope, *The Complete Medicinal Herbal.* New York: Dorling Kindersley, Inc., 1993.

Orellana, Sandra L., *Indian Medicine in Highland Guatemala: The Pre-Hispanic and Colonial Periods.* Albuquerque: University of New Mexico Press, 1987.

Programa de Salud Herberea Corporacion Metodista SEDEC, *Medicina Natural.* Concepcion, Chile: SEDEC, 1998.

Queens Botanical Garden, *Harvesting Our History: A Botanical and Cultural Guide to Queens.* Flushing: Queens Botanical Garden, 1998.

Roeder, Beatrice A., *Chicano Folk Medicine from Los Angeles, Calif.* Berkeley: University of California Press, 1990.

ltes, Richard Evans, and Robert F. Raffauf, *The Healorest: Medicinal and Toxic Plants of the Northwest ia.* Portland: Dioscorides Press, 1990.

Seaford, C. E., *Folk Healing Plants Used in the Caribbean.* Trinidad: A.L. Falaah Productions Ltd., 1988.

Severynse, Marion, *The American Heritage Stedman's Medical Dictionary.* Boston: Houghton Mifflin Company, 1995.

Sheldon, Jannie Wood, Michael J. Balick, and Sarah A. Laird, *Medicinal Plants: Can Utilization and Conservation Coexist?* Bronx: The New York Botanical Garden, 1997.

Soustelle, Jacques, *The Daily Life of the Aztecs.* New York: Macmillian Company, 1961.

Taylor, Leslie, *Herbal Secrets of the Rain Forest.* Roseville: Prima Publishing, Inc., 1998.

Weiner, Michael, *Weiner's Herbal.* Mill Valley: Quantum Books, 1990.

Wren, R. C., *Potter's New Cyclopedia of Botanical Drugs and Preparations* (rev. ed.). Saffron Walden, UK: C.W. Daniel Company, Ltd., 1988.

SCIENTIFIC AND MEDICAL PERIODICALS

Abad, M. J., et al., "Antiinflammatory Activity of Some Medicinal Plant Extracts from Venezuela," *Journal of Ethnopharmacology* 55 (December 1996), pp. 63–68.

Algeria, Daniel, et al., "El Hospital Invisible: A Study of Curanderismo," *Archives of General Psychiatry* 34 (November 1977), pp. 1354–1357.

Almeida, Edvaldo Rodrigues de, et al., "Antiinflammatory Action of Lapachol," *Journal of Ethnopharmacology* 29 (May 1990), pp. 239–241.

Appelt, Glenn D., "Pharmacological Aspects of Selected Herbs Employed in Hispanic Folk Medicine in the San Luis Valley of Colorado, USA: I. *Ligusticum Porteri*

(Ohsa) and *Matricaria Chamomilla* (Manzanilla)," *Journal of Ethnopharmacology* 13 (1985), pp. 51–55.

Bhakta, T., et al., "Evaluation of Hepatoprotective Activity of *Cassia fistula* Leaf Extract," *Journal of Ethnopharmacology* 66 (1999), pp. 277–282.

Bhargava, S. K., "Antifertility Agents from Plants," *Fitoterapia* LIX, 3 (1988).

Bird, H. R., and I. Canino, "The Sociopsychiatry of Espiritismo: Findings of a Study of Psychiatric Populations of Puerto Rican and Other Hispanic Children," *Journal of the American Academy of Child Psychiatry*, 1981, pp. 725–740.

Bose, Aruna, et al., "Azarcon por Empacho—Another Cause of Lead Toxicity," *Pediatrics* 72 (July 1983).

Caceres, Armando, et al., "Diuretic Activity of Plants Used for the Treatment of Urinary Ailments in Guatemala," *Journal of Ethnopharmacology* 19 (March–April 1987), pp. 233–245.

———, "Plants Used in Guatemala for the Treatment of Gastrointestinal Disorders. 3. Confirmation of Activity Against Enterobacteria of 16 Plants," *Journal of Ethnopharmacology* 38 (January 1993), pp. 31–38.

———, "Plants Used in Guatemala for the Treatment of Respiratory Diseases. 1. Screening of 68 Plants Against Gram-Positive Bacteria," *Journal of Ethnopharmacology* 31 (February 1991), pp. 193–208.

Chamber, Bruce A., et al., "Initial Trials of Maytansine, An Antitumor Plant Alkaloid," *Cancer Treatment Reports* 62 (March 1978), pp. 429–438.

han, Ashok K., et al., "A Review of Medicinal Plants ng Anticonvulsant Activity," *Journal of Ethnology* 22 (January 1988), pp. 11–23.

Chen, Zheng-Ping, et al., "Studies on the Anti-Tumour, Anti-Bacterial, and Wound-Healing Properties of Dragon's Blood," *Planta Medica* 60 (1994), pp. 541–545.

Council on Scientific Affairs, "Hispanic Health in the United States," *Journal of the American Medical Association* 265, 2 (January 9, 1991), 248–252.

Damodaran, S., and S. Venkataraman, "A Study on the Therapeutic Efficacy of *Cassia alata*, Linn. Leaf Extract Against *Pityriasis versicolor*," *Journal of Ethnopharmacology* 42 (March 1994), pp. 19–23.

DiStasi, Luiz C., et al., "Screening in Mice of Some Medicinal Plants Used for Analgesic Purposes in the State of São Paulo," *Journal of Ethnopharmacology* 24 (September 1988), pp. 205–211.

Eisenberg, David M., et al., "Trends in Alternative Medicine Use in the United States, 1990–1997," *Journal of the American Medical Association* 280, 18 (November 11, 1998), pp. 1569–1575.

Erdelmeier, C. A. J., et al., "Antiviral and Antiphlogistic Activities of *Hamamelis virginiana* Bark," *Planta Medica* 62 (1996), pp. 241–245.

Filho, Valdir Cechinel, et al. "Isolation and Identification of Active Compounds from *Drimys winteri* Barks," *Journal of Ethnopharmacology* 62 (1998), pp. 223–227.

Freiburghaus, F., et al., "Evaluation of African Medicinal Plants for Their In Vitro Trypanocidal Activity," *Journal of Ethnopharmacology* 55 (1996), pp. 1–11.

Garrison, Vivian, "Doctor, *Espiritista* or Psychiatrist?: Health-Seeking Behavior in a Puerto Rican Neighborhood of New York City," *Medical Anthropology* 1, 2 (Spring 1977).

Gene, Rosa M., et al., "Anti-inflammatory and Analgesic

Activity of *Baccharis trimera*: Identification of its Active Constituents," *Planta Medica* 62 (1996), pp. 232–235.

Gilbert, Benjamin, et al., "Activities of the Pharmaceutical Technology Institute of the Oswaldo Cruz Foundation with Medicinal, Insecticidal and Insect Repellent Plants," *An. Acad. Bras. Ci.*, 71 (1999), pp. 265–271.

————, "The Official Use of Medicinal Plants in Public Health," *Ciencia e Cultura: Journal of the Brazilian Association for the Advancement of Science* 49, 5/6 (September–December 1997), pp. 339–344.

Gonzalez, J., et al., "*Chuchuhuasha*—A Drug Used in Folk Medicine in the Amazonian and Andean Areas. A Chemical Study of *Maytenus laevis*," *Journal of Ethnopharmacology* 5 (1982), pp. 73–77.

Gotteland, Martin, et al., "Protective Effect of Boldine in Experimental Colitis," *Planta Medica* 63 (1997), pp. 311–315.

Hernandez, Lesbia, et al., "Use of Medicinal Plants by Ambulatory Patients in Puerto Rico," *American Journal of Hospital Pharmacy* 41 (October 1984), pp. 2060–2064.

Hirano, Toshihiko, et al., "Effects of Stinging Nettle Root Extracts and Their Steroidal Components on the Na+, K+-ATPase of the Benign Prostatic Hyperplasia," *Planta Medica* 60 (1994), pp. 30–33.

Ibrahim, Darah, and Halim Osman, "Antimicrobial Activity of *Cassia alata* from Malaysia," *Journal of Ethnopharmacology* 45 (1995), pp. 151–156.

Kang, Jaw-Jou, and Yu-Wen Cheng, "Effects of Boldine on Mouse Diaphragm and Sarcoplasmic Reticulum Vesicles Isolated from Skeletal Muscle," *Planta Medica* 64 (1998), pp. 18–21.

Kassler, William J., et al., "The Use of Medicinal Herbs by

Human Immunodeficiency Virus–Infected Patients," *Archives of Internal Medicine* 151 (November 1991), pp. 2281–2286.

Lichius, Johannes Josef, and Carola Muth, "The Inhibiting Effects of *Urtica dioica* Root Extracts on Experimentally Induced Prostatic Hyperplasia in the Mouse," *Planta Medica* 63 (1997), pp. 307–310.

Lozoya, X., et al., "Spasmolytic Effect of the Methanolic Extract of *Psidium guajava*," *Planta Medica* 56 (1990), p. 686.

Lutterodt, George D., "Inhibition of Microlax-Induced Experimental Diarrhoea with Narcotic-like Extracts of *Psidium guajava* Leaf in Rats," *Journal of Ethnopharmacology* 37 (September 1992), pp. 151–157.

Lutterodt, George D., and Abdul Maleque, "Effects on Mice Locomotor Activity of a Narcotic-like Principle from *Psidium guajava* leaves," *Journal of Ethnopharmacology* 24 (September 1988), pp. 219–231.

Marsh, Wallace W., and Mary Eberle, "Curanderismo Associated with Fatal Outcome in Child with Leukemia," *Texas Medicine* 83 (February 1987), pp. 38–40.

Marsh, Wallace W., and Kae Hentges, "Mexican Folk Remedies and Conventional Medical Care," *American Family Physician* 37 (March 1988), pp. 257–262.

Marwick, Charles, "Growing Use of Medicinal Botanicals Forces Assessments by Drug Regulators," *Journal of the American Medical Association*, February 22, 1995, p. 607.

Mota, M. L. R., et al., "Anti-inflammatory Action of Tannins Isolated from the Bark of *Anacardium occidentale* L.," *Journal of Ethnopharmacology* 13 (1985), pp. 289–300.

Mudgal, V., "Studies on Medicinal Properties of *Convolulus pluricaulis* and *Boerhaavia diffusa*," *Planta Medica* 28 (1975), pp. 62–67.

Muller, Klaus, et al., "Potential Antipsoriatic Agents: Lapacho Compounds as Potent Inhibitors of HaCaT Cell Growth," *Journal of Natural Products* 62, 8 (1999), pp. 134–135.

Ness, Robert C., and M. D. Wintrob, "Folk Healing: A Description and Synthesis," *American Journal of Psychiatry* 138, 11 (November 1981), pp. 1477–1481.

Oga, Seizi, et al., "Pharmacological Trials of Crude Extract of *Passiflora alata*," *Planta Medica*, 1984, pp. 303–306.

Oliveira, Maria Gabriela M., et al., "Pharmacologic and Toxicologic Effects of Two *Maytenus* Species in Laboratory Animals," *Journal of Ethnopharmacology* 34 (1991), pp. 29–41.

Pachter, Lee M., "Ethnomedical (Folk) Remedies for Childhood Asthma in a Mainland Puerto Rican Community," *Archives of Pediatric and Adolescent Medicine* 149 (September 1995), pp. 982–988.

———, "Home-Based Therapies for the Common Cold Among European American and Ethnic Minority Families," *Archives of Pediatric and Adolescent Medicine*, November 1998, p. 1083.

Padma, P., et al., "Effect of the Extract of *Annona muricata* and *Petunia nyctaginiflora* on Herpes Simplex Virus," *Journal of Ethnopharmacology* 61 (1998), pp. 81–83.

Paiva, L. A. F., et al., "Gastroprotective Effect of *Copaifera langsdorffii* Oleo-resin on Experimental Gastric Ulcer Models in Rats," *Journal of Ethnopharmacology* 62 (August 1998), pp. 73–78.

Petersen, Alyss F., "Alzheimer's Research Advance," *Genetic Engineering News* 19, 10 (May 15, 1999).

Rabe, Tonia, and Johannes van Staden, "Antibacterial

Activity of South African Plants Used for Medicinal Purposes," *Journal of Ethnopharmacology* 56 (1997), pp. 81–87.

Rao, V. S. N., et al., "Antifertility Screening of Some Indigenous Plants of Brazil," *Fitoterapia* LJX, 1 (1988).

Risser, Amanda L., and Lynette J. Mazur, "Use of Folk Remedies in a Hispanic Population," *Archives of Pediatric and Adolescent Medicine* 149 (September 1995), pp. 978–981.

Rizzi, Renato, et al., "Mutagenic and Antimutagenic Activities of *Uncaria tomentosa* and Its Extracts," *Journal of Ethnopharmacology* 38 (January 1993), pp. 63–77.

Roman-Ramos, R., et al., "Anti-hyperglycemic Effect of Some Edible Plants," *Journal of Ethnopharmacology* 48 (August 1995), pp. 25–32.

Ruiz, A. Ramos, et al., "Screening of Medicinal Plants for Induction of Somatic Segregation Activity in *Aspergillus nidulans*," *Journal of Ethnopharmacology* 52 (1996), pp. 123–127.

Sharma, S. S., and Y. K. Gupta, "Reversal of Cisplatin-Induced Delay in Gastric Emptying of Rats by Ginger (*Zingiber officinale*)," *Journal of Ethnopharmacology* 62 (1998), pp. 49–55.

Simoes, C. M. O., "Antiinflammatory Action of *Achyrocline satureioides* Extracts Applied Topically," *Fitoterapia* LIX, 5 (1988).

Soulimani, Rachid, et al., "Behavioral Effects of *Passiflora incarnata* L. and Its Indole Alkaloid and Flavonoid Derivatives and Maltol in the Mouse," *Journal of Ethnopharmacology* 57 (1997), pp. 11–20.

Souza-Formigoni, Maria Lucia Oliveria, et al., "Antiulcerogenic Effects of Two *Maytenus* Species in Laboratory

Animals," *Journal of Ethnopharmacology* 34 (1991), pp. 21–27.

Speroni, E., and A. Minghetti, "Neuropharmacological Activity of Extracts from *Passiflora incarnata*," *Planta Medica*, 1988, pp. 488–491.

Trotter, Robert T. II, "Folk Remedies as Indicators of Common Illness: Examples from the United States–Mexico Border," *Journal of Ethnopharmacology*, 1981, pp. 208–220.

Tubaro, A., et al., "Evaluation of Antiinflammatory Activity of a Chamomile Extract After Topical Application," *Planta Medica*, 1984, p. 359.

Ubillas, R., et al., "SP-303, an Antiviral Oliogomeric Proanthocyanidin from the Latex of *Croton lechleri* (Sangre de Drago)," *Phytomedicine* 1 (1994), pp. 77–106.

Vasquez, Beatriz, et al., "Antiinflammatory Activity of Extracts from *Aloe vera* Gel," *Journal of Ethnopharmacology* 55 (1996), pp. 69–75.

Villarreal, M. I., et al., "Cytotoxic Activity of Some Mexican Plants Used in Traditional Medicine," *Fitoterapia* LXIII, 6 (1992).

Yamahara, Johji, et al., "Cholagogic Effect of Ginger and Its Active Constituents," *Journal of Ethnopharmacology* 13 (1985), pp. 217–225.

Zayas, Luis H., and Philip O. Ozuah, "Mercury Use in Espiritismo: A Survey of Botanicas," *American Journal of Public Health*, January 1996, p. 111.

MEDICAL ABSTRACTS VIA MEDLINE

(Available through the National Library of Medicine of the National Institutes of Health)

Abad, M. J., et al., "Antiviral activity of Bolivian plant extracts," *Gen Pharmacol* 1999 Apr 32(4):499–503.

Applewhite, S. L., "Curanderismo: Demystifying the health beliefs and practices of elderly Mexican Americans," *Health Soc Work* 1995 Nov;20(4):247–253.

Banerjee, S., and A. R. Rao, "Promoting action of cashew nut shell in oil in DMBA-initiated mouse skin tumour model system," *Cancer Lett* 1992 Feb 29:62(2):149–152.

Bolarinwa, Raji Y., "Antifertility activity of *Quassia amara* in male rats—in vivo study," *Life Sci* 1997;61 (11):1067–74.

Burkhard, P. R., "Plant-induced seizures: Reappearance of an old problem," *J. Neurol* 1999 Aug, 246(8):667–70.

Chavis, H., et al., "Friedelane triterpenoids from *Maytenus macrocarpa*," *J Nat Prod* 1998 Jan; 61(1):82–5.

El Sayah, M., et al., "Action of polygodial, a sesquiterpene isolated from *Drimys winteri*, in the guinea-pig ileum and trachea 'in vitro,' " *Eur J Pharmacol* 1998 Mar 5;344(2–3):215–21.

Emery, D. P., and J. G. Corban, "Camphor Toxicity," *J Pediatr Child Health* 1999 Feb;35(1):105–06.

Gebhardt, R., "Antioxidative and protective properties of extracts from leaves of the artichoke (*Cynara scolymus* L.) against hydroperioxide-induced oxidative stress in cultured rat hepatocytes," *Toxicol Appl Pharmacol* 1997 Jun; 144(2):279–86.

———, "Inhibition of cholesterol biosynthesis in primary cultured rat hepatocytes by artichoke (*Cynara scolymus* L.) extracts," *J Pharmacol Exp Ther* 1998 Sep;286(3):1122–8.

Goerge, J., and R. Kuttan, "Mutagenic, carcinogenic and cocarcinogenic activity of cashew nut shell liquid," *Cancer Letter* 1997 Jan 15:112(1):11–16.

Hammer, K. A., et al., "Antimicrobial activity of essential oils and other plant extracts," *J Appl Microbiol* 1999 Jun: 86(6):955–90.

Hayashi, K., et al., "Antiviral activity of an extract of *Cordia salicifolia* on herpes simplex virus type 1," *Planta Medica* 1990 Oct;56(5):439–43.

Iyer, R. P., et al., "*Brunfelsia hopeana* I: Hippocratic screening and antiinflammatory evaluation," *Lloydia* 1977 Jul–Aug;40(4):356–60.

Kamtchouing, P., et al., "The protective role of *Anacardium occientale* extract against streptozotocin-induced diabetes in rats," *J Ethnopharmacol* 1998 Sept;62(2): 95–9.

Katsasou, A., et al., "Frequency of incidents reaction to the European standard series," *Contact Dermatitis* 1999 Nov, 41 (5):276–9.

Kong, Y. C., et al., "Antifertility principles of ruta graveolens," *Planta Medica* 1989 Apr:55(2):176–8.

Lopez, Abraham A. M., et al., "Plant extracts with cytostatic properties growing in Cuba," *Rev Cubana Med Trop* 1979 May–Aug 31 (2):97–104.

Mendes, G. L., et al., "Anti-hyperalgesic properties of the extract and of the main sespuiterpene polygodial isolated from the barks of *Diymys winteri* (Winteraceae)," *Life Sci* 1998;63(5):369–81.

Montoya-Cabrera, M.A., et al., "Fatal poisoning casvo by oil of epazote, chenopodium graveolens," *Gac Med Mex* 1996 Jul–Aug:132(4):433–7.

Ramos Ruiz, A., et al., "Screening of medicinal plants for induction of somatic segregation activity in *Aspergillus nidulans*," *J Ethnopharmacol* 1996 Jul 5;52(3):123–7.

Ruppelt, B. M., et al., "Pharmacological screening of plants recommended by folk medicine as anti-snake venom—I.

Analgesic and anti-inflammatory activities," *Mem Inst Oswaldo Cruz* 1991;86 Suppl 2:203–5.

Spainhour, C. B. Jr., et al., "A toxicological investigation of the garden shrub *Brunfelsia calcyina* var. *floribunda* (yesterday-today-and-tomorrow) in three species," *J Vet Diagn Invest* 1990 Jan;2(1):3–8.

Suarez, M., et al., "Use of folk healing practices by HIV-infected Hispanics living in the United States," *AIDS Care* 1996 Dec;8(6):683–90.

Swanston-Flatt, S. K., et al., "Glycogemic effects of traditional European plant treatments for diabetes. Studies in normal and streptozocin diabetes mice," *Diabetes Res* 1989 Feb;10 (2):69–73.

Tratsk, K. S., et al., "Anti-allergic effects of oedema inhibition caused by the extract of *Drymis winteri*," *Inflamm Res* 1997 Dec; 46(12):509–14.

NEWSPAPERS

Brody, Jane E., "Herbal Remedies Tied to Pregnancy Risks," *The New York Times*, March 9, 1999, p. F1.

Cheng, Mae, et al., "Keeping Well in a New World," *Newsday*, September 28, 1997, pp. A6–7.

DeStefano, Anthony M., et. al. "Remedies from Home," *Newsday*, October 1, 1997, p. A5.

Ochs, Ridgely, "A Second Opinion," *Newsday*, February 15, 1999, p. A13.

Sanchez, Ray, "Well Armed: Faith, Family in Mind, 'El Duque' Shines," *Newsday*, October 23, 1999, p. A5.

GOVERNMENT DOCUMENTS

Form S-1 Registration Statement: Shaman Pharmaceuticals, Inc. Securities and Exchange Commission, Washington, D.C., September 2, 1999.

NEWS RELEASES

ProteoTech, Inc., "Researchers pinpoint structure within proteoglycans critical to enhancement of beta-amyloid protein fibril formation that occurs in Alzheimer's disease," April 16, 1999.

————, "Researchers report that a natural plant derivative from the Amazon rain forest in a rodent model inhibits the deposition of beta-amyloid deposits associated with Alzheimer's disease plaques," April 16, 1999.

Shaman Pharmaceuticals, Inc., "Shaman.com Announces Expansion Into New Markets For Normal Stool Formula," June 27, 2000.

CONSUMER PERIODICALS

"Herbal Rx: The Promises and Pitfalls," *Consumer Reports,* March 1999, pp. 44–48.

WEB SITES CONSULTED

The American Botanical
Council
http://www.herbalgram.org

The Centers for Disease
Control
http://www.cdc.gov

The Baylor College of
Medicine
http://www.bcm.tmc.edu

The Food and Drug
Administration
http://www.fda.gov

Medicinal Herbs of St.
George Village Botanical
Gardens of St. Croix
http://www.ecani.com/st.
george.botgar/medhrb.htm

Milestones
http://www.milestones.org

Mothernature.com
http://www.mothernature.com

The National Institutes of
Health
http://www.nih.gov

*The New England Journal of
Medicine*
http://www.nejm.com

The New York Academy of
Medicine
http://www.nyam.org

The New York Botanical
Gardens
http://www.nybg.org

The Raintree companies
http://www.rain-tree.com

Shaman Pharmaceuticals,
Inc.
http://www.shamanbotanicals.
com

The World Health
Organization
http://www.who.int

Acknowledgments

Since this project started from scratch, there were numerous people who provided assistance to me along the way in what turned out to be an eye-opening journey. I want to thank them all at this time.

While rummaging through some magazines at the library of the New York Botanical Garden, my wife, Susan, found a listing for a conference on ethnobotany that was to be held in September 1999 in Costa Rica. Symposium organizer Ronald Chaves invited me with open arms, saying he would be honored by my presence, and I traveled to San José, Costa Rica, for what proved to be an informative week as a participant at the International Symposio Ethnobotany. The papers presented and the informal talks provided me with a great deal of background material that proved useful in the writing of this book, and for that I thank Professor Chaves and his coorganizer, Dr. Alaine Touwaide.

I also want to thank the various participants in the symposium who provided me with useful information: Emanuela Appetiti, Dr. Bradley Bennett, Margalis Bittner, Doris Burtscher, Dr. Paola Capone, David Crandall, Dr. Nina Etkin, Dr. Mildred Garcia, Dr. Felicia Heidenreich, Maritza

Hoeneisen, Christine Kabuye, Dr. Ruth Kutalek, Dr. Irm-
gard Merfort, Dr. Daniel Moerman, Dr. J. du Plooy, Dr. Armin
Prinz, Luis Proveda, Adriana Quiros, Dr. John M. Riddle,
Solveig Schrickel, Dr. Vassiliki (Betty) Smocovitis, Lucy
Swart, John Weeks, and Dr. Zohara Yaniv. In particular, I
would like to single out Kattia Rosales of the Instituto Nacional Biodiversidad Inbio in Costa Rica for providing me
with insight into her country's medicinal plants and also for
providing me with useful documents.

Closer to home, my wife, Susan, patiently guided me
through the intricacies of using Microsoft Word and saved
me from despair when things were not going right with the
computer. Susan's understanding and support, particularly
given all of the other things that occupied her attention during the time I was writing, helped me a great deal. My father, Michael DeStefano, also spent time recalling his
younger days in East Harlem.

At the New York Botanical Garden in the Bronx, Karl
Lauby and Michael Balick provided me with important materials and leads. In Manhattan, Antonio Mora and his associates Lisa and George Vargas gave me insight into the
botánica culture. From Hawaii, *curandera* Elena Avila gave
me guidance on her healing art. At Shaman Pharmaceuticals, Lisa Conte and Steven King were generous with their
time and attention, as was Dr. Alan D. Snow of ProteoTech,
Inc., and Gordon Cragg of the National Cancer Institute, as
well as Nancy Jeffery at the New York City Department of
Health.

Two friends from Romania, Virginia Farcas and Carmen
Firan, were helpful in recalling their childhood experiences
with herbal medicines. I also appreciate the patience of
my colleagues at *Newsday* in Queens, particularly assistant

managing editor Les Payne, who accommodated my schedule to allow me to write this work.

Lastly, I want to thank my agent, Laura Dail, her assistant, Francheska Farinacci, and my editors at Ballantine, Cathy Repetti and Allison H. Dickens, for their encouragement in carrying out this project.

About the Author

ANTHONY DESTEFANO is an assistant city editor of *Newsday* in Queens, covering criminal justice and legal affairs, as well as the changing face of New York through immigration. He previously worked at the *Wall Street Journal*. DeStefano was part of the *Newsday* team of reporters who won the 1992 Pulitzer Prize. He is a graduate of Ithaca College, Michigan State University, and New York Law School.